EIGHT THEORETICAL APPROACHES IN DANCE-MOVEMENT THERAPY

Edited by

Penny Lewis Bernstein, Ph.D., DTR

Antioch New England Graduate School

KENDALL/HUNT PUBLISHING COMPANY

2460 Kerper Boulevard, Dubuque, Iowa 52001

Library of Congress Catalog Card Number: 79-84222

ISBN 0–8403–2026–4

Printed in the United States of America

B 402026 01

To our students and clients

Theorists seek to come into the presence of a god at a distant shrine. They hope to achieve this presence in part as a direct result of effort, discipline, faithful progress (Giorgi, 1975, p. 256).

Contents

Preface

The purpose of this book is to begin to provide the field of dance-movement therapy with a theoretical body of knowledge through the scrutiny of the major frames of reference utilized by movement therapists in the practice of psychotherapy. In addition, the essence of each theoretical model has been gleened and commonalities formulated into a fundamental conceptualization of dance-movement therapy.

Students, practitioners, and professional colleaques have continued to pose basic questions regarding the fundamental basis of dance therapy. All agree there is a foundation which is germaine to all approaches, yet these postulates had not been sufficiently documented nor articulated. So dance therapists, such as myself continue to respond somewhat cautiously, "yes, there is a body of knowledge in dance therapy" and "yes, movement therapy has its own unique view which distinguishes it from other forms of psychotherapy."

What that view is has begun to be answered in this book. The profession is growing and will continue to evolve. Stipulating some of the basic premises will not stagnate the field as some may believe, but rather provides a firm groundedness in what is so that dance therapy can step beyond, elaborate and flourish.

And what of the intuitive process? Will documenting a body of knowledge curtail the richness of that universal pool? I feel quite the contrary. Rather, conscious conceptualization will serve to shed light, provide a focus and give form to the intuitive. Basic Truth, if it is in fact Truth, will maintain its integrity whether it emerges from the great ocean of the unconscious or is formulated by the cognitive within wo/man's psychology.

Penny Bernstein

Acknowledgments

To those who ponder the questions and seek the answers, the editor of this book is indebted. For these individuals have facilitated the ever emerging relationship to the theoretical body of knowledge in dance-movement therapy.

Diana Beattie, Cathy Conkling, Pamela Patton, and Sheila Hunt contributed their energy to the cover.

This editor would also like to acknowledge the supportive critiquing and counseling of Dr's Rollo May, Donald Polkinghorne, and Laurel Milberg.

Section I

INTRODUCTION

Chapter 1

HISTORICAL PERSPECTIVE IN DANCE-MOVEMENT THERAPY

But what is dance therapy?* Surely a statement of conceptualized theory cannot be made without first knowing what the field involves and where its roots lie.

Dance As Healing Ritual

"Every dance is and gives ecstasy" (Sachs, 1963, p. 49). Movement ritual has allowed individuals since the beginnings of civilization to bridge the gap between themselves and their universe. It affords a vehicle for their expression and transmission of fear, sadness, anger, and joy in the quest for survival and the meaning of live. One of the earliest drawings discovered was executed on cave rock by Paleolithic man depicting a figure dancing in a buffalo skin. This use of the mimetic is found in Sachs' classification of image dances. It is one of two categories he employs to describe the cross-cultural forms of dance ritual. Within this type, the essence is based on what is experienced through sensual perceptions. Thus the pervading belief systems are contingent upon the capacity to cause the metaphorical to become real. *Similia similibus* is the fundamental message. Animals, enemies, or gods, are personified in the image dancer often to the point of possession. Unconscious frenzy is the norm particularly when the dancer receives the spirit of a god. This phenomenon occurs particularly in the dances of Siva, Osiris, Dionysus, and the many gods of Mexican and American Indians. "And out of the deified dancer is formed retrogressively the beautiful conception of the dancing god who creates the world and keeps it in sacred order" (Sachs, 1963, p. 79).

Survival of a more fundamental nature engrossed much of the pre-industrial individual's energy. Imitative dance was used as a prime vehicle for the allaying of feelings of powerlessness and the transmuting of possible potential anxiety into a creative releasing form which permitted wo/man to feel that s/he did, in fact, have some control over personal subsistence whether s/he be hunter, fisher, or farmer. The Eskimo dances in which the hunters become their victims, the African Masai's lion dance, and the turtle dances of Samoa are examples of the hunter's attempt to insure game for his family. Animal dances also serve to receive the magical power, physical strength, and/or courage of the animal, and as a means to propitiate the slain animal's spirit.

Likewise many fertility dances have been performed throughout wo/man's relationship to agrarian survival. Much of these rituals are based on the unifying relationship between human fertility and the seeding and fruition of the soil. Rites of passage also often have imitative qualitities which serve the purpose of instruction to the pubescent, those to be married, to give birth, or to pass from this world to the next.

*Dance therapy is defined as the psychotherapeutic use of movement as a process which furthers the physical and pyschic integration of an individual (American Dance Therapy Association, 1975).

Those dance rituals in which the roots of therapy are most clear, however, are those of the "imageless dances" in which the primary goal is one of attainment of a transcendental ecstasy. Here the dancer's focus is inward toward the eventual release of ego. The outer world is replaced by exhilaration. The circle, a universal symbol of totality (Jung, 1964) is frequently the structural motif. Hypnotized by the repetitive rhythmic movement action and supported by the enclosure of the circle, wo/man surrendered to frenzy often merging with others. From the trance dancing in Bali and Africa and the Dervishes in Moslem East Asia, religious rapture and transcendence allowed wo/man a release from mundane anxieties and conflicts and liberation from the frustrations of humanity.

The Greek chorus or choreia (coming from the root chara, "joy") is akin to this form of dance. It was used in rites of passage, religious exhilaration, and as an integral part of their dramas. In the Dionysian cult, ecstatic liberation is the prevailing theme. The Greek women became mad, and were summoned by the gods. Leaving their families, they climbed the snow capped mountains; and there, intoxicated, raved for days.

Often the ritual dance is primarily carried out by one individual: the medicine man or shaman. S/he engages in a transcendental experience to aid his/her tribe in receiving messages from the spirits, assisting in rites, and healing the sick. It is to the latter that this discussion now focuses. "We may say that at the dawn of civilization dancing, religion, music, and medicine were inseparable. The dance of medicine man, priest, or shaman belongs to the oldest form of medicine and psychotherapy in which the common exultation and release of tensions was able to change man's physical and mental suffering into a new option on health" (Meerloo, 1960, p. 24). An example of this process is shown in Katz's phenomenological elucidation of the healing ceremonies of the !Kung tribesmen of the Kalahari Desert (Katz, 1976). These people, led by their healer, engage in "healing dances" for the treatment of every possible malaise. Individual, family and community problems are all worked through in this manner. During the dance, "n/um," a primal energy said to be found in fire, originates in wo/man's corporal center of gravity and at the base of the spine. Through pelvic movements the dance activates the "n/um" driving it up the torso to the base of the skull where a transcendance of "!kia" occurs. At this point the healer can begin to cure. The individual's sickness is drawn into the healer through his fluttering hands which are placed at the site of the illness. At one point his whole body is encircling his patient. Once the disease is in the healer's body, he exorcises it by shaking his hands and shuddering. Katz states, "Healing nurtures each person's emotional and spiritual growth as well. The dance heals the whole person" (Katz, 1976, p. 85).

The Vedda of Ceylon and the Ute of North America also utilize a spiritual medicine man who transcends to the gods to do battle and insure the well-being of their people. Here again, dance is seen as the most primary vehicle for this purpose (Sachs, 1963, p. 63).

What relevance does the history of ritual dance have to dance therapy? Some of the pioneers in the field feel it's vital to the full understanding and richness of movement therapy. Espenak writes, "The rediscovery of trance-dance and ecstasy has given birth to a new awareness in dance therapy" (Espanek, 1975, p. 103). Bartenieff feels that "part of the struggle for ordering our lives in thought, feeling, and action, can be facilitated through the crystallization of such moments of revelation and discovery into group ritual dance" (Bartenieff, 1975, p. 118). Finally, Bernstein and Bernstein reintroduce concepts from ritual process into a view of group dance-movement therapy which promotes dance therapy as the new ritual process of the modern alienated Western culture (Bernstein, Bernstein, 1973).

History of Dance Therapy

Although dance as ritual continued to play a vital role in the native cultures of the Americas, in Asia, and Africa a sharp decline emerged at the end of the twelfth century in its presence in Europe. There theologians feared its potential inherent power. Even the Renaissance dances were limited to stylized court entertainment. This superficial trend continued until the beginnings of the twentieth century when Isadora Duncan emerged barefoot and emotive on the stages of Europe, and modern dance was born.

The development of psychology has as part of its roots Darwin's *The Expression of Emotions in Man and Animals.* Although it was published in 1873, it required a twentieth century mentality to begin to comprehend some of his ideas. Freud, the uncontested father of psychoanalysis, opened the door; but it was not until his students, Adler, Reich, and Jung, began their work, that the resurgence in an awareness of the whole person and bodily movement began to be reasserted. It was Wilhelm Reich who turned his psychoanalytic chair around and looked at the patient's body. He analyzed not only what the client repressed but how he repressed it somatically as well. Reich developed an elaborate character analysis system based on the defensive armoring of the body and the process of regaining adaptive mobility. Specific movement exercises were designed to contact blocked tense areas of the body allowing affective expression and release.

Carl Jung's development of the techniques of "active imagination" affording the patient a vehicle for expressing unconscious material also paved the way for movement therapy. Jung believed that it is vital for the individual to contact and understand the symbolic information from the unconscious. Once personal material is stripped from the complexes, their archetypical core provides a means for individuation and the experience of Selfhood. He utilized dreams and artistic processes as direct avenues into understanding what was "meant to be" for the person. For this purpose, Jung had used dance either as direct expression or through the "dancing out of one's dreams" (Jung, 1961).

Dance therapy emerged gradually with a firm grounding in the worlds of dance and psychology. It was in the fifties that Mary Whitehouse, an American European trained creative dance teacher who, after Jungian analysis, began to draw connections between the authentic movement expressions of her students and the flow of symbolic material being shared at the end of her class. Individuals who had no desire to dance professionally continued at her studio. Their work with her had had a profound impact on their lives. Her shift into the hithertofore undelineated role of dance therapist was thus a gradual and thoughtful evolution.

On the East Coast, another name had already emerged a decade earlier into the forefront—that of Marian Chace. Trained by the Denishawn School, Chace began a dance studio in the Washington, D.C. area utilizing a creative improvisational dance format. Many individuals attended her classes with the sole idea of personal expression in mind. Among these persons were private patients of some leading psychiatrists in a large federal hospital, St. Elizabeth's. As they heard and observed the effects of these classes on their patients, they decided in 1942 to invite Miss Chace to work with them on the drugless back wards of St. Elizabeth's. From twenty-five years of training all ages in dance and improvisation, her sensitive eye and creative intuitive process were highly honed. She worked with the back ward non-verbal populations and met them where they were. This entailed her moving with them in a synchronistic empathetic manner which let the individual know, "I accept and want to be with you where you are."

Chace writes, "Dance Therapy, in making use of the basic form of communication, offers the individual a means of relating himself to the environment or to people when he is cut off in the majority of areas by the patterns of his illness.

"His meaningful though bizarre movements become understandable and acceptable to others as people relate themselves to him on the basis of the emotions expressed through dance action. As his feeling of isolation and his fear of a lack of understanding are reduced, he is able to put aside autistic expression to an increasing degree, and this in turn, seems to enable him to enter a group and function within it in a manner that is satisfying both to the patient himself and to others in the group" (Chaiklin, 1975, p. 137).

There are three other prime sources in the development of dance therapy in America: The first is Trudi Schoop who, with an improvisational development touch, paralleled much of Chace's work on the West Coast. Liljan Espenak's european training, integrated into Adlerian depth psychotherapy provided an approach to the retarded as well as the functionally impeded. The other source emerged from the followers of Rudolf Laban. Laban devised a system of observation and notation of movement entitled effort-shape* which focuses on how an individual moves. The Dance Notation Bureau founded in New York by Irmgard Bartenieff provided a center where the emerging dance therapists could learn a movement language for evaluative, communicational, and testing purposes. She had brought science into dance therapy.

By 1964, a small number of dance therapists were ready to become a professional body. With Marian Chace as their president, seventy-three people formed the American Dance Therapy Association the following year. Their goals were to denote and promulgate professional standards and to afford a vehicle for communication among hithertofore isolated dance therapists (Schmais, 1974, p. 9).

Yearly conferences provided a forum for learning. Through presentations other professionals began to be known. Among these were Elaine Seigel who brought a new respect for the integration of psychoanalytic theory and movement therapy; and Diane Fletcher, who, utilizing Bion's conceptualizations of the individual and the therapeutic process, brought a slightly different view of a psychodynamic approach to body work.

Maslow's humanistic influence began to emerge more forcefully in the late sixties along with a resurgence of the use of dance toward a transpersonal integration. Barbara Govine reflects this trend.

Many dance therapists have been influenced by Fritz Perls' Existential Gestalt Therapy and have begun to expand their conceptual and technical repertories. Penny Bernstein delineates this integration.

By far the majority of practicing dance therapists in psychotherapy in a (1978) study carried out by the American Dance Therapy Association ascribe to one or more of the theoretical frames of reference reflected here by key proponents. These approaches may serve specific or various populations of individuals but they all provide a conceptual basis for the vitalization of dance-movement therapy.

*Effort denotes the dynamics of energy in space, force, and time; and shape relates to the actual form a movement takes in space.

Chapter 2

THEORY BUILDING IN DANCE-MOVEMENT THERAPY

"A theoretical frame of reference is a set of interrelated, internally consistent concepts, definitions, postulates and principles that provide a systematic description of and prescription for a practitioner's interaction within his domain of concern" (Mosey, 1970, p. 5).

Concepts

Concepts then are the basic foundation for theory building. In the case of a human art-science such as dance therapy, these concepts are propositional in nature as empirical validation is difficult to come by when relating to human beings and their experience. A concept is defined here as an abstraction which represents a particular class of situational events and/or behaviors (Ford and Urban, p. 36). There are various hierarchial levels of event-classes that can be delineated from the specific to the more general (see Figure 1, p. 8).

Another form of grouping is depicted in Table 1 (p. 8). Here level one represents observable behavior and a sequence of responses to an event. Level two begins to describe the pattern of events with labels such as helplessness, fear of rejection, and a "can't do it" attitude. Level three describes a larger constellation of behavior: oral character, which implies that the first level sequence is one of many recurring events.

Postulates

Postulates consist of the relationship between concepts either of a correlative or cause and effect nature. Jung's idea of synchronicity is an example of related events that occur together where causality is not necessarily present. On a more concrete level, locked knees often accompany tense gluteal and external rotator muscles as part of an orally fixated character (Lowen, 1971).

Habitual repetitive movement patterns linked to a reliving of past events as though they were present will result in a diminished adaptability and lessen the awareness of the uniqueness of each moment. Cause and effect is reflected here.

The following references will be employed in this chapter:

Mosey, Anne. *Three Frames of Reference for Mental Health.* New Jersey: Charles B. Slack, Rb, 1970; Ford, Donald and Urban, Hugh. *Systems of Psychotherapy.* New York: John Wiley and Sons, Inc., 1967; Burton, Anthony. *Operational Theories of Personality.* New York: Brunner-Mazel, 1974; Hall, C.S. & Lindsey, G. *Theories of Personality.* (2nd ed.). New York: John Wiley, 1970.

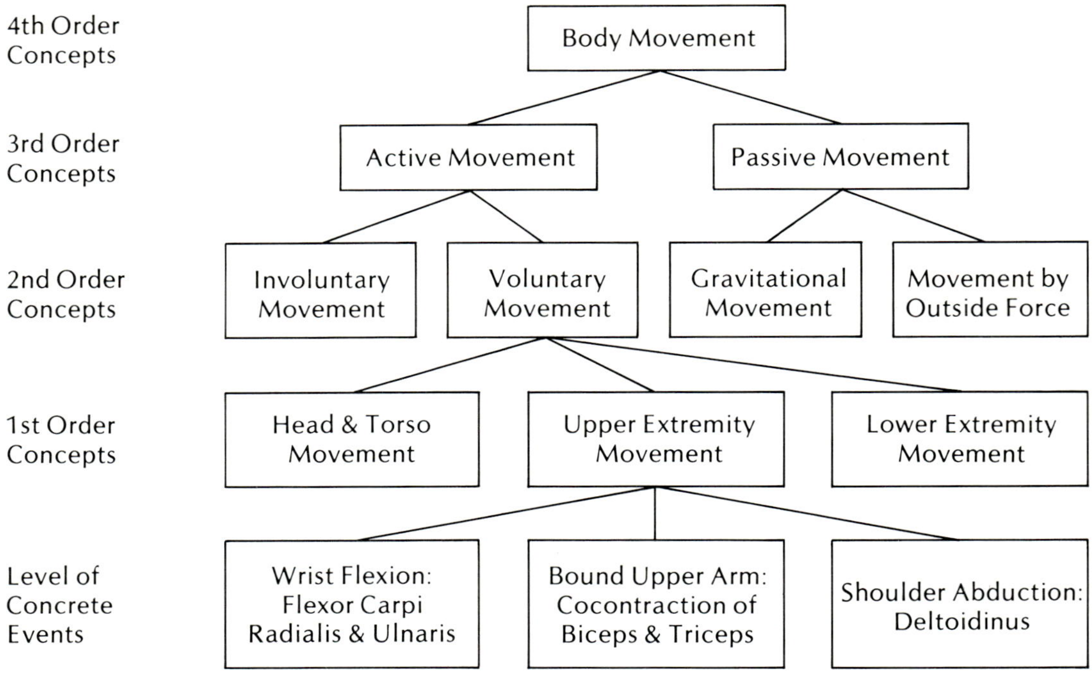

Figure 1. Concepts and their Relationship within a Hierarchical Agreement (Ford & Urban, 1967, p. 37)

Table 1

Levels of Conceptualization (Ford & Urban, 1967, p. 67)

Level Three:	Oral Character
Level Two:	Unable to reach out to satisfy needs Feels helpless, hopeless Needs basic nurturance
Level One:	Body Attitude Upper torso: Collapsed and Closed Arms: Limp and lifeless Chin: Extended Breathing: Belly movement only Interactional Patterns: Friend offers postural embrace, Individual stands lifeless, Then briefly gestures with forearms, Retreats

The major forms of postulates are:

Assumptions discuss untestable relationships such as in the case of the two fundamental premises upon which the study of behavior rests: (1) "the behavioral stream occurs in a lawful fashion, and that not only are the events which go to make it up orderly, but also that this order is potentially identifiable through careful and systematic analysis," and (2) "every behavioral event must be presumed to be related to some antecedent, concurrent, or consequent events in some way" (Ford and Urban, p. 78).

Hypotheses are concerned with observable and, therefore, potentially testable events. The field of dance-movement therapy is actively engaged in the testing of its propositions.

Propositions delineate that area of postulates which tie concepts together in an orderly logical system. They provide an understanding based on hierarchial levels of behavior from which either inductive or deductive inference can be made.

Empirical propositions refer to the relationships between observable events and are linked with testable hypothetical formulations.

Formal propositions, like the assumptions, implicit in their development deal with levels of conceptual abstraction.

Theory

Theory of psychotherapy, then, relates a set of procedures for changing behavior. Procedures which have organized logical concepts provide interrelated building blocks and reflect internally consistent propositional statements.

Outline of Questions

A theory of Dance-movement Therapy must, at some level, respond to the following questions:

1. How is the individual viewed?
2. How is the health-dysfunction continuum viewed?
3. How is dance-movement viewed?
4. How is therapy viewed?
5. How is dance-movement therapy viewed and what are its goals?
6. What is the method of observation and evaluation of the health-dysfunction continuum?
7. What is the therapeutic process, i.e., what are the conditions and sequence for change?

1. How Is the Individual Viewed?

Concepts, along with empirical and formal propositions regarding the individual need to be delineated within the context of the frame of reference. Intrapsychic structure, mind-body relationship, and body movement all need to be, in some way, articulated. Basic human development and postulates regarding learning should be discussed. The individual in relation to the primary other, groups, and his/her culture may also be relevant. A few of the theories speak to wo/man's relationship to the transpersonal as well. In each case, postulates may come from one theory or from the integration of information from dance, psychology, physiology, neurology, kinesiology, sociology as well as the study of more esoteric healing practices from other cultures.

2. How Is the Health-dysfunction Continuum Viewed?

Delineation of the behavioral nature of health is discussed and utilized as a global goal or direction in therapy. The empirical and formal propositions concerning dysfunction draw the therapist into more explicit attention as to what is to be treated by the application of the frame of reference. Distinctions regarding each continuum provide a clearer guide for use in treatment and its evaluation.

Dysfunction may be defined utilizing various levels of conceptual abstraction such as lack of ego boundaries or may be stated in terms of body movement such as habitual non-adaptive neutral flow or an inability to maintain grounded contact with the floor (Bernstein, 1974).

Here the distinction between symptom and pathology (maladaptation) should be made.

Pathology is defined as "that which the frame of reference is designed to alter" while *Symptoms* "are those behaviors which point to or indicate dysfunction" (Mosey, 1976, p. 11). Typically a constellation of symptoms are employed to describe a dysfunction. Important to note here is that one approach's symptom may be another's dysfunction. Blockage of body flow is considered a dysfunction by Reichians, to psychoanalytic therapists, it is considered a symptom. In either case, this behavior should disappear as a continuous orientation to the environment.

3. How Is Dance-movement Viewed?

Postulates concerning the medium by which "dance" therapy distinguishes itself from other forms of psychotherapy must also be elucidated. Dance-movement is limited to the experience of an individual's body in motion. Since movement is an essential factor for all life forms, it is an element of being-in-the-world that is continuously present from birth to death. Breath flow and body posturing are also included in this area as the former entails a change however minute in body shape, and the latter involves some form of muscle contraction no matter how disaligned in order to maintain verticality.

4. How Is Therapy Viewed?

Concepts which describe what psychotherapy does and for what purpose are explicated here. It is generally assumed that therapy is viewed as a professional relationship between a trained person (dance therapist) and another (client, patient) who is in some way dysfunctional for the purpose of movement toward more healthy functioning. Each view, of course, reflects the theoretical horizon in which it is couched. Each frame of reference has its own way of looking at the individual-being-in-the-world and the change in this relationship.

5. How Is Dance-movement Therapy Viewed?

The psythotherapeutic use of movement toward the physical and psychic integration of the individual provides a skeleton upon which the various approaches will sculpt their uniqueness.*

6. What Is the Method of Observation and Evaluation of the Health-dysfunction Continuum?

A theoretical formulation delineates the methods that are utilized to observe the behavior which reflects a dysfunction-health continuum. Evaluation is a process of identification of the

*American Dance Therapy Association, 1975.

point at which the individual is along the continuum at a given time. Evaluation may or may not include interpretation of observable behavior depending on the basic foundational concepts of the approach.

7. What Is the Therapeutic Process?

Here postulates regarding change in the form of internal and external, environmental conditions are sequentially discussed. Step by step process provides both descriptive and prescriptive material. An attempt has been made to generalize the treatment so that the process is germaine to work with all the dysfunction-health continuums with which the model is employed. Thus, this last perspective on the theoretical approach provides a structural guide through the therapeutic journey—a libretto, if you will, for the art of dance therapy.

For the purpose of this examination, the contributors responded to the following questions through three possible horizons:

Genesis speaks to the therapists own personal evolution toward the utilization of the particular theoretical frame of reference she utilizes.

Some made use of an organic method of exploring the practice of their dance experiences with others. This exploration ranges from studio work with students to actual clinical practice. Others focused on their growing awareness and understanding of the continuum of health and dysfunction through the body-movement repetoires of their students/clients/patients. Exploration of various theoretical premises provided a vehicle for others to bridge cognitive conceptualizations with the observable experience. Ecclectic, but internally consistent, theoretical approaches emerged often with unique systheses resulting in propositions germaine to dance therapy. Still others seeing the effectiveness of a specific model and its direct congruence with the movement therapy process adopted the existent theoretical frame of reference. In these cases, specific relevant concepts and propositions are usually emphasized more while others become less important.

These evolutionary methods for theoretical formulations have been discussed separately; however most of the contributors' experiences reflect their multiple usage.

Theoretical Model is the section which speaks specifically to the delineation of conceptual material. Fundamental concepts are defined and discussed in the light of dance therapy application. Theoretical formulations delineate the method of observation and evaluation of the health-dysfunction continuum and the therapeutic process. The role of the dance therapist within the treatment process is related, frequently elaborating on areas such as transference, countertransference and the use of touch and "moving with" the individual.

Case Study as a method of revealing the frame of reference by means of application is the final approach to the elucidation. In each case, one individual's journey in Dance-movement Therapy is described. The therapeutic process is discussed in the light of the model employed. In some instances the total process is related, in others a specific segment of time in the individual's psychotherapy or a particular theme is highlighted. Some individuals have been viewed within the context of a group while others rely solely on the one-to-one relationship.

A bibliography with specific references in each approach is provided for further in-depth reading.

Section II

THE THEORETICAL FRAMES OF REFERENCE

Chapter 3

THE CHACE APPROACH TO DANCE THERAPY

*Sharon Chaiklin, DTR**
*Claire Schmais, Ph.D., DTR***

Genesis***

This passage of time allows me to sort out learning from feelings in my relationship with Marian Chace. She was an intense and complex woman; and in her presence, one could not always keep these separate. When I went to visit Chace at St. Elizabeth's Hospital in Washington, D.C. in 1964, it was with a sense of excitement and anticipation. Chace's writing had stirred something within me. For years I had been searching for a way to express my interest in dance and people. Her account of her work seemed to suggest an answer; but as yet I didn't know what it was.

That first day we eyed each other and then agreed that I would come weekly. I would start as a participant observer in her groups and some of those led by Catherine Hamilton (Pasternak). I proceeded to follow Chace around, observe, participate and ask my endless questions. I quickly learned that there were no observers, but only participants in every group. I was totally involved.

Gradually I was allowed to take over parts of sessions and finally to lead when Chace was elsewhere. I was also priviledged to observe and aid in the annual patient productions she directed. After a year's time, I got her "permission" to pursue a job at another hospital.

Marian Chace taught but she never quite shared the whole. Upon leaving St. Elizabeth's, my reaction was a bit like an adolescent. There was so much more to learn and maybe the "old lady" didn't really know all that much. Experimenting, learning from others, evolving, maturing, learning some more and integrating has been a continual process since that time. However, the more I've learned the more I understand what I first but dimly absorbed from Marian.

Those single, tersely written sentences of Miss Chace's seem even more profound; some of which I am seeing for the first time because I just now understand them. The knowledge and

This paper was jointly written and the authors are, therefore listed alphabetically. The authors apprenticed with Chace at St. Elizabeth's Hospital, Washington, D.C. over a years' time (1964–1965) and Claire Schmais took her course at Turtle Bay Music School, New York City, in March 1960. By observing and questioning Chace, the authors were able to absorb, understand and apply her methods of using dance in therapy. She did not easily share her vast knowledge and experience, nor provide a coherent theoretical framework, but if one was determined to learn, Chace was generous and patient in her support.

*Sharon Chaiklin is a dance therapist at Gundry Hospital, Baltimore and has a private practice in Columbia, Maryland. She trained with Marian Chace at St. Elizabeth's Hospital, Washington, D.C., 1964–65. She has been active in ADTA since its conception and is a field work supervisor in Goucher's graduate program.

**Claire Schmais is an Associate Professor and Coordinator of the Dance Therapy Master's Program at Hunter College; she is an Adjunct Assistant Professor at Cornell University, Medical School; she is Certified in Effort-shape and has a Dance Therapy practice with children and adults.

***Genesis related by Sharon Chaiklin.

ideas that others share can be taken, but they must be incorporated and made usable through the addition of one's own way of seeing and responding to the world. It is hard for me to separate what was first Chace and what I have added to it. It has become mine and it is a gift from her for which I shall always be deeply indebted.

There have been many times over the last few years that I truly miss Marian Chace; miss her because she would have known just how to handle a hostile lady I'm facing, and I want her advice; miss her because I have reached the point where I could discuss and question a point more in depth and would love her opinion; miss her because I might now be able to respond to her in a way which is more equally shared and therefore would lessen her burden.

I think I am closer to understanding. I can resolve many problems myself. I learned this too from Marian Chace.

Theoretical Model

Marian Chace, during the forties and fifties, pioneered the use of dance as therapy. Through revising, refining, and expanding her original ideas, she gradually evolved principles and methods of practice that are now viewed as the theoretical basis of dance therapy. However, she never presented her material in a systematized manner. Her papers were always designed to meet the immediacy of a lecture, conference or publication and thus were limited by the demands of the specific context. Though it is evident that much thought and scholarship went into the development of her work, Chace's existing papers do not contain any references or bibliographies. However, in reading all of her writings, the basic concepts are there to draw from—concise, unadorned and as relevant and profound as when first conceived (Chaiklin, 1975).

Chace began to explore the therapeutic use of dance while teaching modern dance classes at her own studio. However, the major expansion of her ideas took shape during her work at St. Elizabeth's Hospital in Washington, D.C. She started working there during the nineteen forties, prior to the extensive use of tranquilizers and other drug therapies. She was able to test her theories with patients who exhibited a wide variety of behavior, such as violence, catatonic withdrawal, hysteria, etc.

Dance Is Communication

Chace's major contributions lay in the recognition and specification of those elements of dance which serve a therapeutic function, and in the development of the interpersonal role of the therapist on a movement level.

The most basic concept and the one from which all others flow, is that dance is communication and thus, fulfills a basic human need. We believe there are four major classifications that encompass the basic principles that Chace used in therapy. Although they are not categorized as such in her writings, we infer that these are the core concepts of her work, by virtue of their repetition and emphasis.

1. Body Action

Chace believed in the intrinsic value of a graceful, coordinated and healthy body. She viewed distortions in body shape and functions as maladaptive responses to conflict and pain. "When the emotions become pathologically oriented, the image becomes distorted" (Chaiklin, 1975, p. 231).

For example, some people bind energy, limit the use of space, disconnect body parts or hold their breath, to guard against feelings such as guilt, aggression and sexuality. Others become hyperactive, exploding in time and space in response to real or imagined fears.

Chace understood that dance actions could help patients feel both relaxed and stimulated, thus preparing them to express emotions. "Since muscular activity expressing emotion is the substratum of dance, and since dance is a means of structuring and organizing such activity, it might be supposed that the dance could be a potent means of communication for the reintegration of the seriously ill mental patient" (Chaiklin, p. 71).

Through dance action, the patient gains motility of the skeletal musculature. Recognizing the body parts, breathing patterns or tension levels which block emotional expression, provide the therapist with clues to the sequence of physical actions that can develop readiness for emotional responsiveness; but it is not merely learning a movement which leads to change. The change occurs when the patient is ready to allow himself to experience the action in his body. There is a close relationship between the integration of postural changes and the shift of psychic attitudes.

> ". . . Only when he is ready for it will it become meaningful to him and effect a change in his body image. . . . You can tell a person to raise their arms, but until they feel it inside you won't get the real lift in the body" (Chaiklin, p. 229).

By understanding the inherent relationship between motility, dance, and emotional expression, the therapist helps the patient to move and be moved.

2. Symbolism

Both the psychotic patient and the dancer make use of symbolic body action to communicate emotions and ideas that defy everyday use of language; however, the intent is different. Whereas the dancer may objectively choose bizarre and exaggerated postures to communicate with an audience, the patient is giving expression to his subjective emotions, conveying in a single moment the complexity and depth of feelings that cannot be put into words.

> "Basic dance* is the externalization of those inner feelings which cannot be expressed in rational speech but can only be shared in rhythmic, symbolic action" (Chaiklin, p. 203).

The universality of these non-verbal symbols can cut across barriers due to illness, age and culture. Schizophrenics, in particular, seem at home with the symbolic language of movement, whereas they often cannot communicate through words, nor benefit from verbal interpretations. The camouflage of the movement symbol makes it easier for these patients to express needs, feelings and desires.

> "Mrs. R. is withdrawn . . . remains curled up in a corner of the room absorbed in her own feelings. . . . Suddenly, after a large circle has been formed, she begins a rhythmic stamping movement of her feet which carries her around the room just outside of the circle of other dancers. As she stamps, she moves her shoulders forward with alternate sharp jerks, reaching with her arms as she chants, in time to the music, about her loneliness and isolation from others.

*"The term 'basic dance' has been coined to differentiate it from the artificial and elaborate forms of dance which depend upon physical 'tours de force' as a means of entertainment, rather than communication" (Chaiklin, p. 219).

> Recently, she suddenly demanded, 'Play that again. It is from 1920 or so.' Asked if she knew the music, she stated, 'It belongs to the time of my beginning.' The music was repeated and she continued to dance throughout the session with unusual intensity. At the close of the hour she relaxed heavily in her chair and in response to the remark said as a question 'You are tired?' She answered, 'Yes, I have just lived twenty years, and now I am here' " (Chaiklin, p. 142).

Symbolism in dance therapy provides a medium by which a patient can recall, re-enact and re-experience. Some problems can be worked through on a purely symbolic level. The dance therapist accepts the symbolic meanings of the patient. Feeling understood leads the patient to continue symbolic statements. The dance therapist not only reacts to the symbolic expressions of the patient but also introduces content. Together they create new symbolic interactions. Since dance and emotional expression share the same neuromuscular pathways, the dance therapist utilizes this linkage by selecting appropriate dance images. For example, to help a patient who is holding back anger, the therapist may suggest the image of chopping down a tree. The strong, direct movements required by this activity may bring to the surface feelings of anger or hostility. The dance actions can also evoke specific memories. Skipping and hopping may lead patients to suddenly recall incidents and events from their childhood.

3. Therapeutic Movement Relationship

Chace discovered how to establish a therapeutic relationship on a movement level. She accomplished this by visually and kinesthetically perceiving the patient's movement expressions. Employing her keen sensitivity and skills, she was able to incorporate the emotional content of the patient's behavior into her own movement responses. She literally expressed "I know how you feel" in movement terms, thus establishing affective, empathetic interactions:

> "Miss H. is dancing, absorbed in her fantasy. She is making use of the music without regard for its color, although she is following the rhythmic pattern. As she moves rapidly about the room, there is no feeling that she is aware of outward space. Her feet barely make contact with the floor; her hands may reach outward, but not into space. She may stretch upward in a grandiose gesture, but it seems strangely disembodied. This creates a feeling of loneliness and removal accompanying whatever other emotions of hate, fear, or need may be the specific theme of her dance.
>
> It would be almost impossible to reach this patient with words. She is absorbed in her own world and she is unable to hear with comprehension. However, it is possible to approach her with a dance that is similar in pattern to her own. The patient will accept another dancer even though the feeling of her isolation remains for a time. The therapist remains with the patient for short periods of time, with a gradual lengthening of these periods. Eventually, the patient usually looks at the other dancer with recognition. Then a quick 'hello' with an answering smile establishes the beginning of a relationship" (Chaiklin pp. 140–141).

Chace entered a patient's world by reenacting the essential constellation of movement characterizing his expression. As she recreated the patient's behavior in her own body, she would sense what was possible and further the interaction by doing similar, broader or complementary movements. She would at various times reflect, expand or complete a patient's tentative movement, thus letting him know that his behavior is understood. By reproducing the significant gesture at the right time and for only as long as the patient would accept it, Chace established trust leading patients to communicate repressed ideas and feelings and to risk new experiences and relationships.

4. Rhythmic Group Activity

Rhythm permeates every aspect of human life. The everyday activities of speaking, walking, working and playing would be chaotic without structure in time. The ebb and flow of the breath and the steadiness of the pulse are very personal human rhythms, yet a group moving together seems to have one breath and one pulse.

Chace often referred to "primitive" dance in her discussions of rhythm:

> "Even primitive man understood that a group of people moving together gained a feeling of more strength and security than any one individual could feel alone" (Chaiklin, p. 54). "I believe that it was not an accident that caused primitive man to make use of music and dance (or rhythmic action) for the purposes of both worship and solidifying group-feeling in a community. It was not accident that the 'magic' of the medicine man (or spiritual leader) was performed through rituals of chanting and body action" (Chaiklin, p. 61).

Chace recognized rhythm as organizing individual behavior and creating a feeling of solidarity and contagion among people. For example, a group rhythm can be shared by patients who have difficulty or a reluctance to follow the spatial design of a movement. As feelings are expressed in a shared rhythm, each member draws from the common pool of energy and experiences a heightened sense of strength and security.

Dance therapy makes use of the most basic movements expressive of emotion. The element of rhythm is added to actions that are used by everyone. Although these movements are often out of a patient's awareness, they are brought into focus through shared symbolic rhythmic action. Chace saw rhythm as a therapeutic tool for communication and body awareness.

These four basic concepts which we have called Body Action, Symbolism, Therapeutic Movement Relationship, and Rhythmic Group Activity, lay the foundation upon which to build a theory of dance therapy.

Psychiatric Setting

Chace developed her work in dance therapy at St. Elizabeth's, a large psychiatric hospital in Washington, D.C. The dance therapy section was part of the psychotherapy branch, and Chace participated in pertinent case conferences and other clinical and educational activities.

Chace worked with all patients; the short-term patients with positive prognoses and the long-term chronic patients on the very back wards. Most sessions were held in ward areas so that patients could choose to enter or leave the session. Patients who were not ready to actively participate with the group could share in the group dynamics from the periphery. A separate dance therapy room allowed patients who were self-reliant to come to their own sessions.

Patients

While most of the sessions were group experiences, Chace also worked individually with patients who needed more direct contact. These patients either found the group setting too frightening, or they were too demanding or disruptive for the group. She would also be referred those patients whose lack of verbal communication, involvement, and participation caused the staff anger and frustration.

Chace characterized the action patterns of three kinds of patients: manic, depressed psychotic and schizophrenic.

The manic patient, as described, charges into space with exaggerated quick movements. Because of his speed and lack of spatial constraint, these movements appear aggressive, but they are rarely directed toward another individual:

> "The ability to use movement as an expression of emotion in a direct way, together with his command of space about him, makes the manic patient an exciting and stimulating dancer. His movements are exaggerated, strong, beautifully coordinated dance motions, but they always appear like expressions of anger, destruction, and despair. He seems to have no mental image of himself as successful, but only as reaching, attacking, and then despairing" (Chaiklin, p. 135).

Though the actions of the depressed patient are not as flamboyant as those of the manic, they are, nevertheless, revealing of inner feelings. Within this category Chace describes two kinds of patients. One is lethargic, slow to respond, indifferent to his environment, yet cognizant of his own reactions.

> "The patients who are experiencing the slowed up state accompanying an emotional depression seem to be more aware of their body responses than the majority of mental patients. They seem to feel an added anxiety, caused by their inability to function in an accustomed way. They will frequently seek dance activity as a constructive means of alleviating their fright and bewilderment" (Chaiklin, p. 136).

The second type of depressed patient deals with his feeling by engaging in endless, unsatisfying activity.

> "The patient who is expressing depression in restless activity seems to feel no reduction of his anxiety in these repetitive actions. Someone may walk twenty-four hours a day, wring hands, or rock in a chair constantly, but his body tensions seem to be as intense at the end of this time as at the beginning, even though there can be no doubt about the feelings being acted out. . . . If left to himself, or met on a purely verbal level, the patient will continue in this type of movement pattern for long periods of time. However, he is often very responsive to movement in rhythm. He can be stimulated to move with a complete change of movement pattern, with an apparent easing of tensions to the point where he can enter into conversation, laugh, and join in group activity, even though on a tempcrary basis" (Chaiklin, pp. 136–137).

The seemingly bizarre movements of the schizophrenic are characterized by withdrawing from space and limiting movements to peripheral body parts: head, feet, or hands. His specific style directly communicates his feelings of fear, guilt, or hostility:

> "He is also revealing through his movement his feelings of helplessness and dependence. It is not strange, then, that he seems to get no relief from anxiety through his posturings when he receives no satisfactory answer from those about him, on a level which he can accept. He seems to be lost in a four-way dearth of communication. The patient is expressing himself verbally in ways which do not communicate for the most part, but saying things directly in ways which are ignored, while those about him are speaking verbally in ways which do not reach him and expressing feelings non-verbally of which they are unaware" (Chaiklin, p. 137).

Goals

Working as a dance therapist, Chace set long-range goals in keeping with the limitations of each individual. Aware of possible directions she might take for each person and for the group as a whole, she structured each session with its own goals, and built a body of experience to serve as intermediary steps in reaching the ideal. Short-range goals changed from moment to moment as relationships developed and patients risked new experiences.

Although we are separating these goals according to the concepts of body action, symbolism, therapeutic movement relationship and rhythmic group activity, it must be realized that there is a continuous and dynamic interrelationship amongst them.

Goals in relation to the concept of the therapeutic relationship:

1. Establishing own identity.
2. Developing trust.
3. Fostering independence.
4. Recreating social awareness.
5. Developing and maintaining own integrity while accepting social influences.

Goals in relation to the concept of body action:

1. Creating a realistic body image.
2. Activating and integrating body parts.
3. Reconstructing the postural gestalt.
4. Becoming aware of inner sensations.
5. Mobilizing energy.
6. Developing mastery and control of body movements.
7. Expanding the expressive range.

Goals in relation to the concept of symbolism:

1. Integrating words, experience and action.
2. Externalizing inner thoughts and feelings.
3. Expanding the symbolic repertoire.
4. Recalling the significant past.
5. Resolving conflicts through action.
6. Gaining insights.

Goals in relation to rhythmic group activity:

1. Sensing own vitality.
2. Participating in shared experiences.
3. Channeling energy within a structure.
4. Being aware of and responsive to others.
5. Promoting interaction.
6. Bonding people with disparate feelings and life styles.
7. Developing awareness of shared feelings and experiences.
8. Developing openness for new learning and acceptance of self.

Therapeutic Process

For Chace, the session began the instant a door was unlocked and she entered the ward. She quietly acknowledged the patients and staff as she passed, weaving a subtle, understated communicational network through her presence. This act of greeting provided her with many clues about the energy and mood of those present. She noted what patients did or didn't do, what was said or the silence itself, the degree of isolation, fragmentation or any other meaningful cues. During the few minutes she took to enter, put down her records and plug in the record player, she could sufficiently assess the mood, tensions and group configurations to determine how best to begin.

If the tenor of the ward was quiet and depressed, she started with soft, slow music to mirror that feeling. If there was a lot of noisy activity and tension, she played an energetic but clearly rhythmic piece to provide a common focus so that individuals could begin to interact in unison with each other. Most often there were many simultaneous emotional overtones, and then Chace began the session with a waltz, which she considered relatively neutral, eliciting few strong emotional reactions, and was at worst "boring." Since she recognized that music stirs many responses due to rhythm, feeling tones and personal memories attached to particular pieces, careful attention was given to the selection of each record.

Whether the patients in the forming of the group were new or past participants, she would start by rapidly picking up and responding to the verbal and body messages of one patient and then quickly move on the next:

> "Although contacts are being made throughout the room on a one-to-one basis between the dance therapist and an individual patient, a number of such contacts may be taking place almost simultaneously. Dance action is so rapid and so flexible that as the therapist leaves one patient momentarily to meet another, the emotion felt and expressed by her may be changed as she turns.
>
> During this period, the therapist has the feeling of building multiple individual lines of communication, none of which may be neglected even momentarily, and all of which will gradually be developed into a group activity, away from herself except as a catalyst" (Chaiklin, pp. 74–75).

She invited participation, but knew how to permit people to say no. All movement was considered valid and expressive within the therapeutic process. Movements indicating hostility, aggression, withdrawal, isolation or any other feelings were equally valued as direct communications. This orientation led her to repeatedly say that dance therapy has to do with working with "the healthy parts" of the personality. Her senses were open to rhythms, muscle tensions, body parts held or used, and the corresponding effects or emotions. She responded to each patient in terms of his particular movement configuration.

> "One patient stands hunched forward, contracted through the abdomen, his whole posture that of a person in terror. The therapist feels the tension within her own abdomen, and using this as a center of action, she develops a tension relaxation dance sequence. The original contraction she feels may be carried into an expansive movement or into some relaxed action, neither of which can be construed as threatening. In either case, it must develop from or be closely related to the patient's own contracted movement" (Chaiklin, p. 73).

Not merely trying to mirror the movement, she used her own body motion to understand and thereby communicate the acceptance and validity of the expression. There is a fine line between empathy on a movement level and mimicry. Mimicry involves duplicating the external shape of the movement without the emotional content that exists in the dynamics and in the subtle organization of the movement.

> ". . . Miss A. was making threatening advances toward the nurses. The physician in charge, who was familiar with the dance sessions, suggested that I dance with her. Although the space available was limited to an aisle between the beds, we danced furiously together. In this instance, I met her hostile movements of attack with similar ones. The patient danced all manner of assaults on me, playing the role of a child in a tantrum stamping her feet and pounding her fists in direct attack, seemingly bent on destroying her partner in the dance. I responded with answering movements of hostility. However, Miss A. never actually touched me, and her actions were always in rhythm to the music being played, as she pantomimed the battle. Later, after she had expended much energy in this way, I sank to the floor in simulated defeat. Miss A. quietly returned to her bed. . . ." (Chaiklin, p. 139).

Chace was aware that answering movement in similar forms dissipates the feeling of apartness, whereas a battle of words increases that feeling. She did not camouflage sadness or pain with false cheer. Empathy meant sharing the essence of all non-verbal expression resulting in what she called "direct communication."

It is possible to examine how the initial contacts evolve into the formulation of a dynamic group. The therapist moves from one patient to another reflecting varied rhythms and moods. She is sensitive to the length of time needed for each person, anticipates the degree of tolerance for closeness, for communication, for touch, and provides closure before the patient feels threatened or needs to make a move to withdraw. This approach is respectful of the patient and allows him to come and go. The therapist is open to physical contact and will extend her hand when she thinks the patient is ready to take it. Initiating touch, however, is the patient's prerogative. Similarly, the distancing and spatial area used is determined by the patient's movement. The therapist moves rhythmically through the room, towards one patient and then away to another, developing a continuity of action and energy based on the emerging movement expression. The flow of movement begins to involve one participant with another. The therapist's presence and movements throughout the room begin to define the space and structure.

Individual boundaries begin to lose clarity and a communal space begins to evolve. When each patient shares a relationship with the therapist and is willing to join with others, a circle is formed. The circle formation permits equal sharing, visual contact among group members and a sense of security in a clearly defined space. Patients can move away and return without disrupting the group. They can be inside it, out of it, peripheral to it and part of it. The circle can grow or contract allowing variations in touch and distance. Leadership can easily be shifted amongst members and people can choose who they wish to follow, to be near, or to avoid.

The circle is the primary structure from which other forms of relating can develop. Its formation signals the beginning of group work. As the circle becomes a secure place, the group members are able to accept a variety of forms such as lines, clusters, and even relatively undefined shapes. Acceptance of variety in structure reflects their changing attitudes and relationships.

The purpose of the first part of the session, the "warm up," is to mobilize the group's capacity for emotional expression and social interaction. The therapist, as a member of the circle, starts the session by initiating a simple movement such as shaking her hands. She performs movements that engage each contiguous joint until the entire body is warmed up. As more body parts are engaged in the action, more of the person is committed to the movement. The pace and energy demands are gradually increased, leading to deeper breathing that becomes integrated with the movement. At the same time, the range of motion toward and away from the body and into the surrounding space makes changes in relationships possible: for instance, one can reach out to someone or pull back. During this period, the therapist successively establishes eye contact with each group member and simultaneously adapts her motions to reflect each individual's unique pattern. She moves simply, rhythmically and repetitively so that all members can join in the action and begin to feel part of the group. The sequence of motion must have some body logic—an easy flow from one part to another which is appealing, esthetically sound and compelling. The dance should be inviting so patients want to join.

After contact is established, the therapist gradually intensifies the patient's movement in order to make them more apparent. Her exaggerating and clarifying the shape and dynamic content of the movement allows the patient to become aware of his own intentions and inclincations to action and inaction. The therapist is the catalyst through which experiences are shared. By displaying her own commitment to emotional expression, she tests the patient's readiness to risk a more direct statement of his feelings. One of our patients who had difficulty in giving or taking was helped to symbolically enact this conflict by simultaneously using one arm to give and the other to take. As the group members share in movement patterns, the patient is given further permission and support to symbolically enact his repressed feelings and desires in a safe place.

The therapist makes moment to moment choices affirming those patients' movements that will lead to healthier functioning. She works with the realities of the moment. Arbitrary patterns are not imposed. Instead, the therapist moves with the patient to help him expand and develop his existing repertoire of actions. This may take the form of extending his ability to be strong in one body part ot experiencing strength in his entire body; moving from a tentative opening and closing to moving toward and away from someone; evolving a partially aggressive movement into a full punch against a specific target; channeling wild thrusts into focused controlled actions.

The therapist also supports spontaneous changes in set movement patterns. Subtle differences are mirrored by the therapist with clarity and direction in order to reinforce the new behavior. This process enables the patient to meet situations with new responses, perhaps with strength he never knew he had or with tenderness he did not dare express.

Tuning in to the affective state is just the beginning of the therapeutic relationship. It is the material out of which the therapist develops a movement dialogue, a group dance whose purpose is self-awareness and emotional growth. By recognizing her own movement inclinations and responses to the group "gestalt," and sensing the developing movements of the group members, the therapist decides what should follow. The therapist makes use of the movement expressions of the group members, builds upon these and encourages spontaneity and continuity of rhythmic interaction. Similar to a piece of choreography, the initial period of development leads to the main body of the session, which may center around one or several themes. Themes are chosen from what has emerged in the movement—feelings of helplessness, mistrust, separation, loss or any one of the many other human feelings or needs:

> "Miss Y. was strongly involved in morbid ideas of death and destruction. She had actually seen death as a solution for severe problems at one time and had killed her husband. Her dances in a creative form led inevitably to this point during one psychotic episode. In combining her creative ideas into a structured form for teaching other people a group dance based on her ideas she was

> able to relate to others for the first time during her hospitalization. The creative dance was the basis for this structuring, but by centering her thinking on the patterns of her ideas for the group to carry out, her interest was aroused in structured forms which were outside of her subjective morbid emotion. Here the creative art was useful, but only with the addition of having to teach and therefore forced her to make her ideas objective rather than a totally direct communication of her morbidity in an exaggerated form" (Chaiklin, p. 216).

Occasionally feelings are verbally expressed, but most often the therapist elaborates on a theme based on a patient's symbolic movement expressions. Her concern is to develop those themes gleaned from the "warm-up" which will allow for the growth and development of each individual and the group as a whole. The quality of movement, spatial arrangements, and rhythms are determined by the intersecting needs of individuals and the group. Each and every movement chosen by the therapist is based on the expressive content of individual group members. These movements are shaped and formed by the therapist in a way which allows the group as a whole to participate. The choices are dependent on the group's readiness to engage in and support a particular group member and his specific emotional expression. During the session, the therapist will have picked up and developed to some degree the movements of each group member.

Though movement is the primary means of intervention, imagery, syntax and voice quality are also used to further the therapeutic process in a dance therapy session. A verbal image often aids in eliciting the quality of movement one is striving to achieve. Asking a patient to walk quickly will evoke one response while asking him to imagine walking on a hot sandy beach will evoke another. The therapist encourages participants to develop imagery related to their own lives and fantasies and to share them with the group.

There is an important difference between eliciting a response by making a demand or by phrasing a question. For example, the question "how tall can you be?" might evoke a variety of answers including, "I can't be tall," whereas the demand "be tall' provides no choice for the patient. Questions are also used to develop simple motions into symbolic actions, i.e., can you push, chop, float, etc.? A further level of verbalization would move the patient from action to interaction, connecting cognition with physical actions. For example, "Who are you punching? What are you chopping?"

The therapist uses her tone of voice to reflect the moods and feelings of the group. She may be soothing or provocative, angry or demanding. The quality of voice reinforces the dynamics of the movement and serves as a link to patients who cannot tolerate eye contact. The therapist's continuous patter helps maintain the group and is especially useful when the movement is difficult to see or do. In addition, on-going verbalization serves to invite insight, identify affect and further interaction. There may be moments when the movement stops and there is just conversation, but more frequently the words are intertwined with the continuous movement, providing for mutual emphasis.

Group members are encouraged to use words and sounds to support their actions. Sometimes connecting rhythms are elicited from the group without the need of music. Patients make noises, clap, stamp, or sing.

The session usually lasts about an hour. The relative length of the initial warm-up, the central development and the ending will vary. There may be sessions where the warm-up stretches on because of the group's reluctance to be committed to any theme or statement until the therapist makes reluctance itself the theme. Other sessions may have a perfunctory warm-up period because there is a surging forth of a multitude of feelings wanting expression.

Closure is particularly important. The work of each session must be resolved so that patients will leave comfortably. This means that there has been a meaningful exchange with each patient and that no one has been left in a vulnerable position. Work and group interaction reaches a natural conclusion. At that point Chace would return to the circle formation, acknowledge each individual and close with simple repetitive communal movements that fostered a sense of camaraderie and well-being.

Summary

Chace evolved a theory for dance therapy practice that has its origins in dance movement. It was through the dance that she found a way to reach psychotic patients. Rather than relying on theoretical models that stress pathology, she sought out motion and health. Her profound understanding of rhythmic movement led her to create a method for contacting and sparking the life force of those afraid and alienated. She was able to break the barrier of isolation and communicate on a peer level with very withdrawn and disturbed people. How well she understood the power of movement with others!

Case Study

Marian Chace focused on group interaction and the resulting dynamics of the group which led to individual growth. A case study might be developed from the perspective of the group itself. Such a study would show how a group, in the process of fulfilling its therapeutic goals, changes its character, structure, thematic material, patterns of relating, and so forth.

Another means of looking at the interactive process is to study the individuals within it. In this study we have chosen to follow the changes of one woman, Rose, who participated in a dance therapy group in a small psychiatric hospital.* We are presenting only those aspects of the group history that clarify how Rose made use of the group as part of her treatment. The treatment model is based on the concepts inherent in the work of Marian Chace.

Background Information

Rose was a voluntary admission to the hospital. She was diagnosed as schizophrenic, chronic, undifferentiated type. Rose, looking older than her years, had an unkempt appearance, gray hair, no facial mobility, and a body which hunched forward. Her history showed early fearfulness and withdrawal. She failed first grade in school and finally left at the end of ninth grade at the age of sixteen. She never managed heterosexual relationships with any success. Her only interests seemed to be her job and driving her car.

She entered the hospital when she was no longer able to work in her clerk's job because of disturbing thought disorders and withdrawal into a fantasy world. "I live in a dream world because reality stinks." Rose was 48 years old at the time of admission, single and living alone. Her IQ was average and she functioned in that range despite her psychosis. There had been a brief admission to a state hospital 16 years earlier. One of the factors involved in her re-hospitalization was her decision to discontinue medication.

Psychological testing toward the end of her hospitalization showed the following:

*This patient was in a group led by Sharon Chaiklin, who is the stated therapist.

"In the unstructured situation presented by the Rorschach and Draw-a-person tests, the patient's thought disorder is even more noticeable and pronounced as are her entrenched defensive postures. She has considerable trouble interpretating reality and she has erected a cautious, evasive, highly guarded wariness to defend against her vulnerability. Ego functions do not seem well integrated even though she can cover up farily well. By not communicating freely and by being cautious, withholding and evasive, she is able to 'function', but the price she pays is severe social withdrawal and isolation from human contact. She is afraid of her fantasies too and tends to suppress that otherwise satisfying and cathartic means of emotional and creative expression. On the surface, she might appear to be almost totally devoid of the ability to fantasize but probably more accurately, she simply is not willing or able to share fantasies with others. This may be actually good for her as her thoughts can be very loose, vague and confused and may put even more distance between her and others if they knew them."

The interdisciplinary team recommended that the treatment goal be helping Rose develop means for reducing her fantasies and increasing her social skills. Because of the long duration of her illness and her entrenched defenses, all that could be realistically expected was that Rose could gain enough control of her psychotic thinking to get back to work. If she could work, she would not be totally isolated and would again have structure to her life. Hopefully, she might also learn to be with others in a satisfying way.

Rose was referred to dance therapy because she needed to develop a clearer body image and skills in relating to others. Her other activities were participating in the general hospital milieu, recreation, crafts, art therapy, and periodic verbal group therapy in addition to drug therapy. Her total length of hospitalization was thirteen months, after which she lived in the self-care unit for a further period. It was possible to know how people in other disciplines were perceiving Rose's behavior from the weekly discussions at the hospital staff meetings. It is this comparison which makes this case particularly interesting.

Rose and Dance Therapy

Rose began a weekly dance therapy session five days after her admission. When she began, she was still in the acute stages of her psychosis, confused and isolated. She seemed to enjoy the sessions but moved with a minimal amount of dynamics; there was occasional lightness and quickness in the movements of her arms and hands. During the first few sessions, she was able to focus on the movements of others and thereby make some changes in her own style. She was unable to identify or make use of her back muscles: her head and torso were sunk, her spatial range limited. For instance, her arms never stretched out fully. Most often she seemed unaware of the space around her.

During one of Rose's early sessions, the group members were particularly cut off from each other. We began to work on becoming aware of the surrounding space and being enclosed within it. People began to push the air in all directions with various body parts, extending their spatial boundaries. Gradually, we cut across spaces and shared space together. The therapist suggested that they use their back and shoulders to push through the space. Many found it difficult to differentiate between movement of the back and of the shoulders. Rose had very little awareness of her back and the space behind her. She participated with the group throughout but remained cut off because of her inability to move through space to the people around her. She was able to lift her torso and head from its very sunken position and stated that "it felt different and good."

During these first weeks, Rose was passive and somewhat depressed but began to get involved in the sessions. She tried to do whatever the group did and her overt thought patterns seemed more appropriate. By the seventh session, she was clearly interacting with the therapist, concentrating, and remembering work of past sessions. However, spatial use remained a problem. Her torso became straighter, but although she was active, her spatial range and coordination did not improve. Each week she became more depressed. The dance therapist's report of the twentieth session states that she is "pulled in, quiet, passive, have to repeat things to her; a hand tremor; no sense of joy, purpose, focus or direction."

It was soon after this that she became physically ill and was taken off all psychotropic drugs. In the following two sessions, though she was present in the room, she did not participate. Upon returning to active participation, she started to show her strength in movement and was getting closer to others. During the twenty-sixth session, she was visually fixated on something in front of her. It was unclear whether or not she was hallucinating. She further restricted her spatial field by visually pinpointing and by not turning or twisting her torso. Her whole body would turn as a unit, maintaining a single alignment. As the therapist commented on her limited use of space, Rose reached out and took the therapist's hand in hers, and initiated a slow rocking motion. The therapist responded to this act of direct communication by saying, "I want to see you. Can you see me?" alluding to the act of seeing both symbolically and literally. Could Rose see someone else and also allow someone to see into her? Rose's eyes became filled with tears. This was the first emotion Rose shared since her admission. Rose and the therapist continued the soft touch of hands while the rest of the group, aware of the importance of this behavior, quietly and supportively grouped around them. Rose opened outward, allowing the group to join hands with them, but immediately thereafter distanced herself from the group members by shrinking into her solitary space.

During the following session, although she was trembling and uncomfortable, she discussed with the therapist the problem that her constantly slipping glasses obscured her vision. Whether or not they were seeing each other became a continuing theme between them.

To maximize these expressions of affect, the therapist requested that drugs continue to be withheld. Recognizing the therapeutic validity of the request, the psychiatrist consented. The dance therapist asked Rose to participate in a second dance therapy group so that she could become more intensively involved. Rose responded positively to the suggestion and at the next session exhibited more active involvement. Her movements, while still limited, were back to the peak of her abilities. She started using the lower half of her body, developing a pattern of shifting her weight from one foot to the other. Her thinking was sufficiently organized to follow a complex pattern and to recall events of past sessions. It was still difficult for her to twist her upper torso. At this time she initiated a movement of her own which she used frequently thereafter, a turning motion with arms up in the air. Her glasses no longer slipped and she said to the therapist, "we can now see each other."

Rose continued to participate actively. As she became more vertically aligned, making better use of her hips and legs, she started to sense her body weight, and eventually her own strength. Her range of movement increased as she moved into new spatial areas and began to use her back with some awareness.

During the thirtieth session, the group was uncomfortable with the hostility of a patient who yelled loudly and refused to participate. To help the group express the hostility, the therapist initiated quick, sharp movements which gradually became slower and calmer. Group members began to rub and pat each other's backs, symbolic of the good feelings they had for each other. The therapist worked on Rose's back as a way of strengthening the relationship through touch. Rose spontaneously returned the back rub and commented that she enjoyed doing that. The following session back rubs were again exchanged, and it was clear that she enjoyed the giving more than the receiving.

As the next few weeks passed, Rose continued to use more energy and showed some sign of being witty. She showed more initiative in interacting with others and began to use the horizontal plane of movement (turning to others) and more varied dynamics. At this time she began to request polka music frequently and responded to the 2/4 rhythms by moving alone or with a partner.

Despite all that was happening in dance therapy, there seemed to be no carry-over into other activities. Nursing staff, recreational aides and the psychiatrist were all reporting a regressed, non-functioning woman. She apparently selected dance therapy as the place to develop a close relationship, express feelings and interact with others.

For no apparent reason, Rose started to regress in the dance therapy sessions to the point of being difficult, hostile and confused. Her thought patterns were again bizarre. She expressed hostility by setting clear limits as to what she would or would not do. At this point the dance therapist conceded that some medication might make Rose more comfortable. She resumed medication which enabled her to function with less confusion. After a month of gradual improvement, the staff began to see the responsive behaviors that had been evident earlier in the dance therapy sessions. She was reported to be verbal, pleasant, and able to do more for herself.

Rose now reversed her use of dance therapy. The sessions became the place to act out the things she was struggling with, her private thoughts, her feelings of isolation and distaste for group experiences. She developed a ritualized walk because "dancing means moving your feet," which consisted of a rhythmic pacing back and forth at a right angle to the group. This continued for six sessions (three weeks). At this point she was not encouraged to join the group, nor to alter her pattern, but instead the therapist praised Rose for doing her own movement so well. She was receptive to this approach, which led to her demonstrating her "turning movement" for the group. She advised them to move their bodies. It was clear that she again had selected dance therapy to work on "other" behavior and needed support to work on her own terms, no matter what they might be.

The following session Rose continued with her walk. When she received support, she added arm gestures. She moved with other individuals in partnership, but the only way she would be part of the whole group was when she was in the center and the circle moved around her. She then did her characteristic rotating movement with her arms held high. The next session Rose joined the group of her own accord and helped form a circle. She remained thereafter, a full and active member of the group, following as well as leading.

Staff began to discuss Rose's leaving the hospital and plans were made to try to have her return to her old job. At this time Rose was placed in a self-care unit where she was far more responsible for her own grooming and care. During this period of indecision, the dynamics of her movements again became limited. She did not use the strength or lightness that she had displayed previously. She began to shrink into herself. During one session the group worked on leaning on each other for the support each could give. Rose was unable to either lean or support. Rose looked well, but she exhibited a great deal of erratic shaking of her legs, body and arms. When asked about it, she answered it was a "rhythm waiting for the music." She was able to deal with this in the sessions by structuring her own involvement in the group, deciding when to be active, when to rest and when to smoke. The group, which had supported her behavior, considered Rose an important member and liked her despite her distancing behavior. Rose left dance therapy after a year's hospitalization to return to her job.

Summary

Dance therapy was the only therapeutic modality that this patient was able to use. For whatever reason, known only to Rose, movement was a non-threatening and supportive therapy which allowed her to "be myself," no matter what that self happened to be at any time. While there were changes in her level of functioning, her total movement behavior did not change very much over time. There was some increase in the use of space, improved coordination, rhythmic responsiveness, and an ability to move with others which was new to her— "I've always danced by myself." There was a close relationship and trust established with the therapist. While one rarely hopes for profound change in the case of a chronic schizophrenic personality, it can be considered a success that Rose was able to reconstitute herself and return to the community. It is not realistic to hope for much more for Rose. It is likely that in this case, dance therapy was a strong contributing factor.

This study illustrates the basic principles of Chace's work. At the body action level, Rose was guided to develop the grounded total body movements that gave her the potential for strength and assertiveness. Symbolic expressions were accepted as direct communications; walking alone represented the need for solitude, whereas her "turning lifting dance" was a statement of well-being. Her symbolic use of seeing was crucial in bridging the gap between solitude and fellowship.

Sharing her feelings through rhythmic movement with the group and the therapist gave Rose the opportunity to gain support, acceptance and the energy to go on. Although dance therapy was not the only influencing factor during her hospitalization, it was clearly the stage on which she could shed defenses and permit her self to be seen.

Bibliography

Chaiklin, Harris, Ed. *Marian Chace: Her Papers*. Columbia: American Dance Therapy Association, 1975.

Chapter 4

REFLECTIONS AND PROJECTIONS: THE SCHOOP APPROACH TO DANCE THERAPY*

*Trudi Schoop, DTR***
*Peggy Mitchell, DTR****

Genesis

On a Monday morning, I stood alone in the hospital's social hall, waiting for my first group of assigned patients. The doctors had trusted my ability to carry out this new program in dance therapy. Right then, I wished I could feel that same confidence. How will the patients react to the sessions? The palms of my hands were tickling again. Why must I be so nervous . . . why so afraid? There was no time to answer myself. An orderly appeared in the doorway, ushering the patients into the hall. Cautiously, they massed together near the entrance . . . waiting. . . .

"Good morning!" My cheerful tone belied my feeling. Something about the way they stood there gave me the impression that they resented having their customary routine interrupted.

"Won't you please come in?" I suggested encouragingly.

Twenty-two patients, categorized as chronic schizophrenics, gradually filtered into the room, bringing with them undercurrents of suspicion, hostility, anxiety, and mistrust. A few examined the piano. Some felt the table, touched a wall. Many circled aimlessly about, staring at the floor, and two men remained at the door, feet defiantly planted. Whatever they were doing, whether these patients were facing me or had their backs turned, I had the sensation of being furtively appraised, of undergoing an unspoken rite of initiation.

"Well, now! I would like very much to tell you who I am and why I am here. Please, will you all sit down in a circle?"

This request, which to my inexperienced mind seemed to be so natural, so simple, presented an unforeseen problem ending in disaster. Every variation of not-sitting-on-the-floor-in-a-circle unfolded before my astonished eyes. One patient draped himself over a chair. One darted across the room and started banging on the piano keys. One stooped down and hid under the table. One rolled himself up in the curtain. Some supported their organized "NO" by lying down, arguing,

*Material for this chapter has been in part abstracted from Schoop, Trudi with Peggy Mitchell: *Won't You Join the Dance*. Palo Alto: Mayfield Publishing Co., 1974.

**Trudi Schoop works in close collaboration with psychiatrists in hospitals and clinics in the Los Angeles area and abroad in Switzerland, France, Germany and Italy. Ms. Schoop does in-service training with hospital staff and provides supervised internship experiences.

***A charter member of the A.D.T.A. and collaborator with Trudi Schoop, Peggy Mitchell has worked as a dance therpist in private practice and in psychiatric hospitals. She is currently studying Consciousness and Energy Fields and their application to the healing process.

asking for a match, giggling, or gazing out the window. But the majority simply retreated to the security of their habitual attitudes, the long-established oblivion of their individual behavior patterns.

I made a few wretchedly unsuccessful attempts to gain their attention. Then I gave up, and concentrated on the few who were on the floor anyway. I sat down with them and began.

"Okay! My name is Trudi. In our sessions together I will include exercises that will strengthen the muscles and make the body flexible. We will have music to dance to, and—"

"Dance!" As if on cue, there was a communal uprising. "Dance," I was told, "is for sissies." . . . "My mother wouldn't approve." . . . "Dance is against my religion." . . . And one woman announced with finality, "My aunt got measles from dancing."

In one offended body, they moved with great dignity toward the door. The orderly shrugged and began to lead them out, and through the commotion I overheard somebody's voice:

"Hey, what ward is she from?"

I was alone again.

Tuesday morning—Again, I heard the patients shuffling down the corridor. Again, I watched them being led in by the same orderly—Mr. Dakin—who looked as tired as his group. The sight of these lackadaisical bodies confirmed my plan for the day's session.

"Today, I would like to work on feelings. Let's show our feelings!" I cried enthusiastically. "And let's begin with being angry. Show me how it is when you are just furious!"

The hall echoed with silence. We stared at each other for awhile.

"I mean . . . show me . . . what are we doing when we are angry? How do we move?"

One thin voice finally broke the deadly hush: "It's not nice to be angry." A second: "I don't move when I'm angry." A third: "I'm not angry, I've never been angry, and I never will be angry!"

"Oh now, come one. It is okay to be angry. We are all angry sometimes, aren't we? I can get very angry!" I was beginning to feel what I said. "I, for instance, stamp my feet. I punch, I shake my fist. Like this!" And I demonstrated these symbols of wrath with all my energy and enormous affect. They liked it.

Encouraged by the first glimmer of interest, I tried to pass the ball. "Okay now! You be angry!"

"Do it again," someone demanded. A chorus of voices joined in, "Yeah, go on, do it again!"

So I repeated my movement study of angriness. Someone laughed. The reaction was heartening, but I knew I couldn't go on and on, entertaining twenty-two patients and an orderly. I had to do better than that. I had promised far more! I had to arouse their feelings! "Stamp! Punch! Hit! Cut! Box! Yell! Be angry . . . furious . . . mad!!" Forty-four eyes stared into faraway spaces. Forty-four arms moved helplessly. Forty-four legs tried to lift their moored feet. Twenty-two minds did not want what I wanted. Twenty-two bodies could not express what they didn't want to feel. Somebody wandered off. Somebody sat down. Somebody gazed out the window, bored, disinterested, listless.

In despair, I again went into action. I hurled my body about in an avalanche of anger. I jumped. I hit. I raced up and down the hall. In sudden turns, I landed an attack, puffing, stamping, spitting fire; I threw myself up in the air and down on the floor in a temper tantrum. Perspiring, my heart pounding . . . I finally stopped.

As I came to, I realized that I had lost my audience. Only two men remained on the scene. One came closer.

"Are you on bennies?" he asked.

Facing the members of my group, I decided to begin with a beautiful swing, soft and fluid. "Let's stand in a semicircle." Their compliance was encouraging. "Now, I'd like you to swing your bodies in any way you want. Invent any kind of a swing. Let your bodies go!"

Nobody tried. I saw fear in one face, confusion in another. What had I said that was so shocking? For me, a swing is a joy. It creates such a marvelously satisfying balance between control and release.

"Think of wheat fields, being blown by the wind, back and forth, up and down . . . or of ocean waves, coming in and going out!" My attempt at imagery also failed. There was no response. What had happened? Somehow, it seemed that I'd touched on dangerous territory.

"Look what I can do!" It was Emma. She bent over and showed me that she could touch her toes without bending her knees. Others began to touch their toes, too.

"I can do push-ups," announced Carl. And he began to demonstrate.

"When I was in the service, I used to do forty jumping-jacks without stopping!" This was Fred. "Come on," he cried "let's do 'em! One-two-three-four, one-two-three-four!"

For the first time, I saw these individuals functioning vaguely as a group. I saw bodies moving. I saw some enthusiasm. Why did they follow Fred and not me? Gradually, the women withdrew from this strenuous masculine competition. They seated themselves close to a wall. One cried. One began to rock. Another picked her teeth.

The session was falling apart again. I must regain control of it somehow. At least there had been some action. Perhaps if I began by animating each body part, and strictly structured every movement. . . .

"Let's see what we can do with our hands!" I called out. "We can move them up and down, side to side, around and around." A few patients started trying to follow the hand motions. "What can we do with our heads?" I continued with more assurance. "They can move up and down, side to side, and round and round and round." Except for the three isolated ones who never deviated from their own movement worlds, all the others were doing something with their heads that looked like rotation. Delighted with this success, I continued eagerly, "And what can we do with our pelvises? They can go side to side, front and back, around and ar—!"

Why did Carl stop? Why were Rosalie and Emma giggling together? What was Walter doing with his back turned? There was a shrill wolf-whistle. Fred was approaching me, his face leering suggestively, his pelvis moving back and forth in blatant sexual invitation. What if Dr. Keermuschel should come in right now? How can I handle this? I wasn't sure anymore. My confidence began to splinter. I ran for the beaters and thrust one into each person's hand.

"Let's all beat a soft waltz rhythm on the floor! Like this: one, two, three, one, two, three!" I made a last desparate effort to unify my fragmented group. But Fred only transferred this stimulated state to this new outlet. Why hit the floor when it was so much more exciting to hit the piano, the curtains, or himself? The other men picked up his lead: beaters became swords; beaters were ripped to pieces; beaters hurtled through the air; beaters chased screaming girls around the room. On the far rim of the chaos, I glimpsed the head of the orderly shaking slowly back and forth. My knees gave way. I sat down hard on the piano bench. My voice sounded faintly in my ears:

"That's all for today."

I began my extended weekend thinking about how miserably I had failed. What fiascos those three sessions had been! I'd just have to phone Dr. Keermuschel and tell him that he'd misplaced his trust in me, that I wasn't qualified to call myself a dance therapist.

I reviewed those sessions again and again. My three hours of mistakes as a dance therapist were becoming more and more valuable. What specific information had I picked up? Exactly what had I learned? I wrote down the results of my ponderings.

1. It is simply impossible to handle twenty-two patients in one class. Six or eight would be plenty, depending on each individual's tendency to cooperate.
2. Each group should consist of patients having more or less the same general disposition:
   Withdrawn patients
   Hyperactive patients
   Patients in farily good contact
   Patients in poor contact
   After a while, there would be the possibility of combining them for purposes of variety and stimulation.
3. If one person's acting-out behavior—his need to "take over" any situation—disrupts the atmosphere of the class, I should take him out and work with him privately until his actions are modified by personal attention.
4. One-to-one sessions would also be necessary for patients out of contact.
5. Oh, and one more thing: the clothes the patients are wearing—or not wearing—are just impossible. Suggest sweat suits for the men, leotards and wraparounds for the women. What a difference that would make!

Now then. Back to my own behavior. What had the patients taught me about myself?

1. I must learn to be flexible.
   I'd planned those sessions too carefully; so carefully that when the patients went off on a tangent, I panicked. I should accept such deviations as a positive indication of the personal expression I am seeking. A new theme could be developed from the patient's digression. My compliance wouldn't mean giving up my objective for that class; it would only represent a detour. If I had encouraged and supported them, if I had joined them in their wish for gymnastics, the patients would have felt that I approved of them and of their contribution. It could have been an active session if I'd grasped the opportunity to expand and vary their own movement theme. At the end, the strenuous exercises might have been readily exchanged for the quiet, swaying swings I'd wanted in the first place. Instead, I had kept myself apart: I had refused to join in on their level; had insisted on my own pre-planned ideas; and had given them no new movement experience. I had rejected their offering.
2. I went too far, too fast.
   "Invent a swing! What an unreasonable request that was! How would anyone know what a dancer means by a swing without first being taught its movement pattern, or shown its quality? And more of this nonsense: "Swing your bodies in any way you want!" Really! I was asking them to make a choice when they didn't even know what they were supposed to be

making a choice about! They were helpless in the face of the freedom I so thoughtlessly demanded.

3. Beware of imagery.
   No one reacted to the images I gave to induce a swing. Maybe they never saw wheatfields in the wind. Maybe they were afraid of ocean waves. Mightn't an image that seems harmless to me be threatening for them? I'd better go easy with this image-giving. Why not let the patients supply their own? I could ask them, "What does swinging remind you of?" Wouldn't that allow each patient to react out of his own experience? Wouldn' it encourage them to be actively involved, to be reliant on their own initiative instead of being passively dependent upon my suggestions? Besides, each person's image-association might give me valuable information about his nature. Who knows? He might even get information about himself!
4. Emotions: Handle with care!
   When I asked my group to display anger, I was met by uncomprehending stares or by various acts of rebellion. Now I realize how naive I was in expecting a person to reveal his emotions, when for years he'd been preoccupied either in suppressing them or avoiding them. "I'm not angry, I never have been angry, and I never will be angry!" That flat statement should have been warning enough. But . . . I know that it's vitally important to bring those submerged feelings to the surface. Ths question is, HOW? When I go back to the hospital, I'll really try to respond to the patient's needs. I'll go very slowly, as if I had a hundred years' time. I'll be open and flexible instead of insistent and domineering. I won't mute my pupils with my own exuberance, or shock them with my theatromania. I won't ask for creative movement before they have acquired a movement vocabulary to be creative with. Nor will I offer freedom until they can cope with it.

One problem still remains unsolved: how can the patient's resistance to emotional expression be overcome? They had refused to acknowledge anger. People stamp when they're mad, so I could use stamps. People punch; we could punch. People kick, slap, claw, pull, push, What would happen if a patient's body repeated such anger-forms, over and over? Would the anger-feeling erupt in spite of his need to conceal it?

Doesn't it seem strange, though, that I would separate action and feeling in order to restore a person's wholeness of being? Well, no, it isn't really so strange. Isn't anyone's state of mind constantly expressed by his body? And, vice versa, doesn't anyone's body-experience influence his state of mind? It doesn't seem to matter whether the process is initiated by the mind or by the body; the two conditions of being continue to interact and reinforce one another.

As for the patients, weren't their mental aberrations mirrored in their physical aberrations? And didn't their bodies' aberrations continue to reinforce the aberrations of their minds?

Of course, these illustrations are oversimplified. Any feeling can be expressed in a thousand different ways. But aren't the physical representations of a feeling based on identical elements of expression which occur reflexively in everyone? Rhythmic patterns, positions, forms, movement designs, degrees of tension, use of space—these principles compose the mutual theme on which the individual performs his own variations. However unique a person's variations may be, we can all recognize the familiar elements that lie behind them. These elements provide the background for human understanding. They are universal; they apply to all people. They are the human expression!

Theoretical Model

These passages from *Won't You Join the Dance?* describe my experiences and ideas of more than twenty years ago. With the passage of time, I find that my original concepts have not drastically changed but that I have changed, grown up a little bit: my perceptions have broadened and sharpened; my enduring love for life has deepened, and my fascination with all of life's expressions has become more profound. In recent years, I have been drawing upon some personal philosophical principles which, I feel, add seasoning and nourishment to my professional service.

By way of prefacing this theoretical model: I feel, realizing my bias, that of all the humans on this planet, dancers are the lucky ones. They are the ones who can be in agreement with the whole procsss of life. They can agree with the changes and surprises that life holds in store for them, and they can agree to any and all of life's colorful expressions. This enthusiastic concordance with life is their strength and their security. Dancers can even feel safe in the midst of crisis because they somehow know that critical changes provide the rhythm and the melody of their presence on this earth within their own particular life span.

Ur Experience

This brings me directly to an idea that I'm most eager to share. I believe that as individuals make their passage through life, they are experiencing two levels of existence simultaneously. The first level, I call the *Ur Experience* "UR" is, of course, a German word. The closest translation I can find in English are such terms as "cosmic," "universal," and "transcendent." The UR experience denotes the eternal, on-going process of cosmic order and harmony. It describes *Energy:* the vital force which keeps the whole universal complex on the move. From the microcosm of the atom to the magnitude of the great, whirling bodies of matter in our heavens and beyond, there exists the ceaseless life-force of the UR Energy.

UR also describes *Time*—time without beginning, time without end, time that continues its on-going, rhythmic flow for no reason that can be comprehended except to continue. And UR describes *Space*—Limitless extensions of space, existing without boundaries far beyond the familiar stars, planets sun, and moon of our galaxy into inconceivable regions.

Humans, by the very nature of the evolutionary process, are linked to the UR Energy, the UR Time-flow, the UR Space. They are indeed, a certain species of living matter conjured up by the combined UR Forces. The UR—incomprehensible as it is—is therefore the primordial portion in each individual. Without the UR, there would be no life at all.

Man's second level of experience is his existence on this earth. He is born into a special human environment—energy-bound, time-bound, space-bound—with a particular pair of parents in association with a particular societal structure, culture, and race. Behind him and before him, lies his evolutionary process on this planet. Thus far in the milleniums, he has progressed from the algae in the seas to the strange and wonderful creature he is today: the creature presently labeled "human." The very quality of being human seems to generate differentiation and individuation. Humanity serves to set each individual apart—one from another. I believe this sense of separateness is common to all and will always be a challenge during human existence on this planet.

But I believe that deep within each human lies a recognition of the UR experience. There are many names for it. Some call it Nature; some call it Paradise; some call it Infinity; some call it God. Whatever its name, the recollection of this level of being permits each individual to have a consciousness of space/time/energy forever unbound. I think that humans can never be fully-rounded and global unless they actualize their UR Experience. They can then be assured that everything that has occurred in man's evolutionary process is within each individual now. Mankind has forgotten nothing—not one thing. Individuals comprehend the eternal Life Force. It is accepted as being so. Individuals say "Yes" to it; "So be it"; "Amen"; or "Right on!"

Let me try to explain this double-track experience in terms of dance. I think that dance expresses both spheres of awareness. Individuals dance within their lifespan here, in their time, in their space, using their individual energies. They feel the security of a floor supporting their moving feet. They feel the muscles of their body stretching and contracting. They feel their strong heart beating—sending blood coursing through their veins. They experience space in all its aspects as their body leaps, sinks, whirls, opens, closes. The rhythmic stamping of their feet in a folk dance, however, is the eternal stamp of man. The muscles that respond to their dance-needs are those that swung the ape through the jungle branches. The energy that carries them through a difficult bit of choreography is the same that mobilized the bodies of the cave man. The lungs that regulate their breathing are but refinements of those acquired by the first sea-creatures who ventured onto the land. The heart of the dinosaur still beats in man's breasts. Dance patterns are created in space with the endless variety of space-forms-in-motion suggested by all living creatures. I honestly feel that a dancer can have the highest comprehension of life-present and life-everlasting. The dancer can recognize and experience the interrelationship of the two existences.

Now, of what real and present value is this sense of connection with the Universal Process? For one thing, the idea of sharing and of having shared a milleniums-long commonality can give each solitary human a sense of security, of belonging, of kinship with one another as each bears, at this point in time, the name of MAN. What's more, the image individuals have of themselves can only reflect the glory of the Universe. If human beings are part of the glory, then are they themselves not glorious? Furthermore, I think it provides them with an innate urge to *go with* life, to become embedded in it, acknowledging peaceably that LIFE IS. Mankind is given the possibility to say "YES" to all of Life's aspects. And lastly, as humans have shared their involvement in the life process, they have acquired fundamental similarities which provide a common ground for mutual understanding, recognition, and communication. Beyond the basic blueprint of human structure and anatomy they have developed a vocabulary that by-passes any language barriers. It is the vocabulary of human expression.

Wholeness

According to my concept of the whole person, all individuals encompass the complete range of every feeling, action, thought . . . from the least to the most, from the smallest to the largest. But it's damn hard to become such a full human! Society usually demands that they become selective: one feeling, action, or thought must be suppressed, another must become dominant. What a toll such discrimination takes on individual personalities! Hospitalized patients demonstrate clearly how devastating the toll can be. It's as if they have become one-sided; locked into a single feeling, all others consigned to oblivion. But are those other facets totally forgotten, rejected, destroyed: I think not. Rather, I believe this form of specilization is arbitrary. The patient has simply chosen to erase the other side of his total coin. But *I* know about the opposite and can slowly, slowly work to return it to his consciousness. Not only do I want to remind him that the other side exists; I want to make him aware that it is actually incorporated in his present extremism. In other words, I believe that opposites are mutually inclusive. One couldn't know about night if one didn't know about day. The fact that an individual can be sad also means that he can be joyful. Kindness contains the understanding of cruelty. Confusion can breed clarity. Loneliness remembers companionship. Intelligence recognizes stupidity . . . "opposites" are merely reverse images of certain states of being.

As a practical example: heaviness includes lightness; these opposing qualities are the Yin and Yang of weight. However, there are people whose heaviness recognizes no lightness. Out of balance, these individuals become one-sided specialists in heaviness. Endless examples of such specialization can be seen: people who are *only* angry, *only* excited, *only* loving, *only* quiet. . . .

It has become increasingly clear to me that man is the only organism on this earth who hides a particular facet of his being; who carries the burden of a secret self. A tree, a flower, a rock, an animal—each shows itself fully. Human beings are the only ones who are selective about what they want to show and what they don't want to show; the only ones who are never entirely present. But I can see the secrecy and the selectivity in a person's body. I can hear it in his voice. This condition is stunningly apparent in the behavior of the schizophrenic individuals with whom I work. And I try, very gradually to bring them back to their totality by tapping into the forgotten sides which still exist somewhere within them and by releasing them from their oppressive secrecy.

You see, I am convinced that every one desperately wants to become what I call "global"; to realize all possibilities. I can recognize this desire in all the people I come in contact with—"sick" or "well." It is not only *my* wish that they experience their wholeness. Each human is driven by a longing to fulfill himself.

Credo

1. Man manifests himself in his body; the body is the visual representation of the total being.
2. Mind and body are in constant reciprocal interaction, so that whatever the inner self experiences comes to full realization in the body, and whatever the body experiences influences the inner self.
3. Whether thoughts and feelings are rational or irrational, positive or negative, split or unified, acknowledged or inhibited, state of mind becomes embodied in the physical being. It is manifested in the body's alignment, in the way the body is centered, in its rhythmical patterns, in its tempo, sounds, use of tension and energy, in its relationship to space, in its potentiality for changes. All these factors determine the body's expression. They affect the way it moves, and moves about.
4. Through the body, man's mind experiences reality. His senses inform his mind of his very being. They tell him how he is, who he is, and where he is. Sight, sound, smell, taste, and touch incite his mental processes.
5. Mind and body are fused by their reciprocal interaction. Their collaboration insures human unity.

Mind-body Interrelationship

The mind-body partnership makes it possible for me to assume that a person can be influenced from either side of his nature. If psychoanalysis brings about a change in the mental attitude, there should be a corresponding physical change. If dance therapy brings about a change in the body's behavior, there should be a corresponding change in the mind. Both methods aim to change the total human, mind and body, which leads me to believe that if the psychotherapist and the dance therapist could be persuaded to join forces, the patient wouldn't stand a chance of maintaining his disturbance.

The transformation of a patient's unfunctional physical distortions presents an enormous challenge, but I must try to reestablish for him a body that will again operate effectively and perform normally, a body that will have a positive, remedial effect upon his mind.

The "Normal" Body

And what do I mean by a "normal" body? Precisely what do I think a body should be like after my dance "treatment"? How would it look, act, and feel? I'll certainly have to clarify my own concept of the body in its most ideal form. I'll need a "body-criterion" which can serve as a basis for comparative evaluation. . .

I envision a being, still in Paradise, living in joyous confirmation of itself, inaccordance with its birth, its life, and its death, and proud of its ability to perpetuate its own image. It is a human form as it was meant to be and to function, in its complete, perfect state-revelling in its breathing, exulting in its motion, beautifully assertive in its total involvement with existence. It is an organic unity wherein mind and body are fused so that the thought is the action and the action is the thought. This being exists in the optimal center of gravity. It moves in balanced relationship between tension and release. Its breath adjusts and flows rhythmically. Its alignment is harmonious, well-centered, ready for change. Its muscle tone is functional, its movement and use of energy effective, and its adaptation to space spontaneous. Ever-curious, its senses are acutely tuned into the sights, sounds, smells, tastes, and textures provided so lavishly by the environment. Delighting in all its possibilities, this body can make itself long or short, wide or narrow, big or small. It can walk, run, jump, leap, turn. It can kneel, crouch, sit, lie down. It can stand on two feet, on one foot-or on its head. It falls, climbs, swims. All such doings can reflect any quality-strong or soft, heavy or light, active or passive and be pleasurably performed in any tempo, from the slowest to the fastest. And the whole marvelous conglomeration can be limitlessly changed, rearranged, organized to suit any human desire, anywhere, at any time.

Such a body wholeheartedly transforms its feelings into appropriate physical manifestations. It shouts in joy, hisses in anger, laughs in amusement, strikes out in hatred, blushes in shame, sobs in grief, relaxes in contentment. It contracts in pain, slumps in exhaustion, stutters in excitement, blocks in fear, yields in love, splits in indecision, and disintegrates in confusion. Constantly and adequately, this body performs its feelings.

Whenever any emotional reaction has been expressed, the ideal body regains its equilibrium. It returns to its point of departure, its home base, which provides the full, unrestricted potential for new experience. Here, any contraction, distortion, or cramp can be released into the most capable, effortless, enjoyable body-feeling. Here, the body will become well grounded if it has flown too high, fluid if it has been blocked, reassembled if it has falled apart, revitalized if its energy has been exhausted. Like a pendulum, this being can swing back and forth between reaction and resolution. Within this stabilizing process, emotion has been given full physical expression; the ideal being has embodied its feeling. Whatever the affective experience, it has taken its course, has been given a form, has been changed, has been resolved. No residue remains to color future encounters. . . . Such was the perfect body I envisioned.

The Conflicted Body

It seems to me that each body I see radiates its own non-verbal message, and that this message represents the sum total of the individual's various characteristics. By means of its unspoken projection, I can sense a personality as being fundamentally open or closed, active or passive, aggressive or defensive. I can see reflections of protest, compliance, acceptance, rejection, affirmation, confirmation, or secrecy. It may convey a strong sense of self or a lack of self-respect. But again, I feel that the most significant of all body-statements is the one that indicates a person's feelings about his own body. He may love it, hate it, or take it for granted. But whatever his prevailing attitude, it will surely influence his relationship to the world around him.

The body broadcasts a person's conflicts as well as his moods. How often he stands at a crossroad in feelings, torn between duty and pleasure, love and hate, should and should not, right and wrong, going or staying. Problematic situations are verbalized quite explicitly: "I'm on the fence." "My feelings are divided." "I'm of two minds on the subject." "I'm really torn."

Disturbed feelings which are so fixed in the body not only reduce and inhibit the physical ability for free performance; they also color any new encounter with life. All future experiences will be influenced by whatever feeling originally created the body's deviation from the functional norm. With pulled-up shoulders, a person responds to any situation by whatever these pulled-up shoulders represent. With tightly crossed arms, a person experiences life "tightly crossed." He is prevented from experiencing spontaneously and realistically. His expectation is fixed.

Identification of the Health-dysfunction Continuum

Human expression, as it is represented by the body, is my source of psychological evaluation. Alignment, centrality, tension, rhythm, use of space: these basic elements of movement and all their related aspects combine to create body-expression. Though these components operate simultaneously and are inextricably interwoven, I do try to separate them for the purpose of body-analysis.

Breathing

Functional breathing enhances the expression of the body by conforming to its feeling: the sharp intake of air in surprise of fear, the heavy expulsion of air in sobs of grief, the deep, rhythmic breathing of love, the full, fluid breathing of joy. Similarly, breathing can adjust in various ways to expedite a person's every action; it adjusts rhythmically to the tempo of his running or walking. It releases with the body in a push or a bend. It sustains an intake of air to lighten the body for a jump or a leap. Breathing actively and effectively assists whatever action or feeling the body undertakes.

Alignment

I feel that it is most significant how a person's body is carried—how he stands on this earth. I believe that a person's body-design should ideally represent his affirmation of being, reflect the highest form of functional existence, realize a neutral, alert attitude from which he can easily act and react. It should indicate a free, adaptable body that is capable of choice and decision, a body with a point of view.

Is a person's carriage straight or crooked? Is his body rooted or aloof? Can he stand on his own two feet, or is he a leaner? Does he feel himself as a harmonious unity, or does he experience himself in bits and pieces? Which bits does he hide? Which ones does he show? These are some of the questions that come to my mind when I'm considering a body's alignment.

Centrality

The center is precisely what the word indicates: the middle area of the human form. It is the center that makes physical and emotional unity possible. Acting as the stabilizer for equilibrium, the compass for orientation, the coordinator for movement, the point of reference that defines physical boundaries, it tells a person where he begins and where he ends. My work has been considerably supported by my belief that the center is the physical equivalent of the human self. As such, it bespeaks the individual's relationship toward his own being and toward the world around him.

Tension

Every one has his own characteristic degree of tension, the one which is the most comfortable and familiar. And it is from this basic level that a person increases or decreases his energy output. Ideally, it represents a condition in which the same amount of tension is equally distributed over the entire body. Whatever the quality of the individual's natural tonicity—soft, strong, light, heavy, fluid, firm—it is unabashedly declared throughout his body. Of course, he constantly leaves this state. Whatever he does, whatever he sees, hears, tastes, touches, smells, whatever he thinks or dreams, his reactions to life cause his tension to increase or decrease. But when the reaction is completed, his tension again becomes harmoniously attuned.

As a person reacts, it becomes more apparent that increasing tension parallels feeling-intensification, just as decreasing tension parallels feeling-abatement. Ideally, the two rise together, reach consummation together, and descend together. This process permits an action to be fulfilled and an emotion to achieve its natural climax. If a person blocks either the feeling or the action in its ascendency, he will never know the gratification of fulfillment. He will forever seek an experience he has denied himself.

Rhythm

Every one is included in the universal rhythm, and I can't believe that there is any one person in this world who is not a part of it. Yet, whenever I introduce rhythmical exercises in my classes, at least one student will desparately explain to me that he never could, and never will be able to follow a beat. But when patients no longer defend themselves against the domination of a given beat, I can open up the rhythmical field. From rhythmical acceptance, we can move to rhythmical disagreement and learn to say "I won't," as well as "I will." The patient can create his own rhythmical combinations within a given structured beat. Again the concept of balance has been presented, between adaptation and individual creation.

Use of Space

The way a body uses space can provide specific information about the individual who owns it. Does a body know where it stands in space? (Has the person a definite point of view?) Can a body maintain a directional course? (Is the person a man of conviction?) Is the whole body unified in the effort to change direction in space? (Can the person make decisions?) Can the body confront, straight-on, the other bodies that share his space? (Can the person face reality?)

I apply every means available to create targets for confrontation, teaching the bodies to "stand their ground," the eyes to look steadily and "take in," the individual to "level" with one another.

Therapeutic Process

I consider the procedure of initiating "full feeling expression" to be truly an artistic process executed by the patient himself.

It is a graudal development that takes place in approximately three separate stages. As therapist, I must first find the appropriate movement means with which my patient can bring his forgotten or hidden feelings out into the light of his awareness. He can then be encouraged to express that secret material in his own authentic movement until he can finally accept the existence of that part of his being. And now the patient alone takes on the responsibility for presenting his subjective, free-floating feeling in an objective, explicit dance form with his body as the instrument for his composition. This esthetic production requires him to organize the forces of both his mind and his body as he does something about himself with himself. As he develops a logical framework for his expression, seeks movement patterns for it, gives it a particular rhythm, a certain step, a special tension, he is gaining the upper hand. His completed production has two positive results: he is now able to experience that feeling without conflict and he can communicate it accurately and realistically. Other people can recognize it. They can react to it. And their response reinforces his own identity.

Relevant to the artistic process of forming: I feel that any work of art, skilled or unskilled, is a creation. And that man himself is a creative being. Those statements bring me right back to my *UR* experience. I think that when man creates form in any of the arts he is drawing on the creative *UR* forces of time, space, energy. Experiences made here in his time are lifted onto another level and the awareness of a higher order is brought to them. On this level, direct communication is possible. Everyone aware of the cosmos within himself, will understand fully.

The dance therapist, knows that the creative forms her patients may achieve will probably be simple and basic. But even a glimpse of the *UR* is sufficient for communication. And communication with other individuals will free them from their isolation. When they can give a surfaced feeling a rhythm, a shape, a direction, a melody, they are sharing themselves with others. They are no longer alone. So what I wish for dance therapists, for me and for our patients is the connection with higher dimensions where secrecy is no longer necessary because the universal past is common to everyone.

The Power of Fantasy

Now I would like to say something about the value of dreams and fantasy in my work with psychotic patients. I believe that what psychosis is is not really known. Instead of defining it, it is only described. In my opinion, the nearest state to psychosis that a healthy person can imagine takes place in dreams and fantasies where, as in psychosis, all things become possible. Fantasies and dreams are *not* psychotic but I think that they are the closest possible link to psychotic experience. All elements of life are differently arranged. Bits and pieces of reality still exist but they are strung together in a distorted way. Laws of time and space are changed. Matter can become transparent. The illogical becomes logical. There are no limitations.

My belief in the positive nature of fantasy has never diminished during my lifetime. I consider it a valuable asset in my work with schizophrenic persons. It allows me the freedom to understand a patient who lives in his dreams where the impossible is possible. To a certain extent at least, I can follow him into those inaccessible regions. I can show him, then, the other side of his world—the physical and practical side. I can connect this side to his fantasies, showing that he can dream with his feet on the ground, again making him aware that both "sides" are present within him; that in this life there is a place for both reality and fantasy. Don't artists move easily between two worlds as they realize a flight of fancy in a poem, a symphony, a sculpture, a dance? I would not want to try to stop the artist from seeing or hearing his fantastic images any more than I would want to prevent the imaginative play of a child. So I feel that rather than suppressing the fantasy of a psychotic individual, I should fly with him for awhile then descend with him for a soft landing on this earth. In giving shape to visions, he will create a work that fuses fantasy and reality.

Every therapist evolves, through experience, her own way of working. I have found that a certain amount of structure helps me to organize my ideas. Whatever theme I have chosen to present runs through a session like a thread, binding consecutive portions together. This kind of reinforcement gives the members of my class a sense of security, of having familiar ground under their feet.

Basic Structure

Idea: *Working with contrasting extremes*

1. Theme: A malfunction of any aspect of the body
   a. Physical representation of the malfunction (how it exhibited in the body?)
   b. Psychological representation of the malfunction (what feelings can be associated with this body?)
   c. Physical and psychological representations of the malfunction's opposite extreme
   d. Working device (correction of the malfunction through exposure to its contrasting extreme)
2. Warm-up
   a. Registering the mood presented by the group, and adapting or adjusting the session accordingly, working to keep it easy-going and non-threatening.
   b. Personal introductions (using names, movement, rhythms, breathing and sounds)
   c. Group contact (interaction in various ways)
3. Instruction: Exercises which increase the body's functional possibilities, while at the same time preparing the body for expression of whatever contract that has been chosen
   a. On floor or standing in place (any dancer's exercises for establishing adequate breathing, strengthening muscles, correcting distortions, and, in general, extending the body's vocabulary)
   b. In space (walks, runs, jumps, hops, leaps, skips, turns—any and all of which movements can be combined in various ways and extended immeasurably by the application of specific rhythms, tensions, qualities, and space patterns)
4. Expression: Connecting the basic theme to life situations
   a. Allowing the patient's body to experience fully his ineffectual position in life
   b. Allowing the patient's body to experience fully the contrasting state of being

5. Creating the functional balance between the two aspects of the theme: Changing the energy level of both extremes, until the body approximates physical and emotional balance.
6. Conclusion: In any movement form, reinforce pleasurably the two aspects of the theme that have been worked with during the particular session, always trying to leave the patient in a state of well-being.

Within this basic structure, I tried to reach certain definite goals:

1. To identify for each person the specific parts of his body that have been unused or misused, and to direct his actions into functional patterns.
2. To establish the unifying interactive relationship between mind and body, between fantasy and reality.
3. To bring subjective emotional conflict into an objective physical form, where it can be perceived and dealt with constructively.
4. To use every aspect of movement that will increase the individual's ability to adapt adequately to his environment and to experience himself as a whole, functioning human being.

Role as Therapist

Now as for my practice in general, I feel that therapy is a dialogue. It includes, "me," who I am and the patient who *he* is. I cannot enforce my "me" on his "him." We are two persons with the equal right to choose the time when we can engage in mutual correspondence. And that, in my opinion, is as it should be. As we work together, I don't want to tranquilize: I want to incite—so that we both become totally involved—intensely preoccupied with living.

Those are my facts. They do seem quite reasonable and practical sitting there in their little black letters. But somehow, there is one very important something missing—the very spirit of dance itself. But there are just no words to impart the measureless sense of joy, the love of live, the enchantment with existence that envelops the dancing human.

Case Study

Alone in my studio one morning, I glanced up to see a black man standing in the doorway. I hadn't heard him arrive; when my eyes accidentally touched him I didn't know whether he was coming in or leaving. He just stood there, strangely weightless and ghostlike, wrapped in deep silence. Finally, carefully, he began to move, circling the room slowly, like a trapped animal. He kept very close to the walls, and his feet seemed to touch the floor only slightly, as if the touch hurt him. I sensed fear with him, all around him—but the feeling of fear itself seemed to have been burnt out of his body. All that remained was the shape of fear, a design of fear.

As I stood, fascinated, and watched Luke edge his way around the room, I became acquainted with his peculiar personal mannerism for the first time. It consisted of three distinct, separate actions, repeated one after the other, always in the same order. To begin, he would suddenly raise both arms in a sweeping arc, which ended with his hands forming precise, devil-like horns on his forehead. Maintaining this devilish or faun-like position, he would make a great, deep bow, then return to his standing posture. For the second movement he would flatten his hands, palms turned down and, using them as if they were sharp cutting instruments, make slicing gestures along his neck. In the final movement he would drop his head on his chest and stroke his hair forward with soft, tender strokes. These three meticulous motions, done in a definite rhythm and with a gentle grace, created an atmosphere of pious humility.

He kept his body in an extreme backward slant: chest caved in, back rounded, head forced down. He bounced when he walked, but it wasn't a happy bounce: the "down" was emphasized rather than the "up." His rigidly held torso rocked back and forth, so that his body looked as if it were saying, "Yes, yes, yes," over and over again. And always, always there were the horns, the cuttings, and the head pattings.

Little by little I tried to interrupt his walking and introduce other movements. He would respond to my suggestions by mutterings, "Oh; oh-oh," giving the one word every manner of inflection and connotation, like an actor searching for the best reading of a line.

"Will you jump with me, Luke, like this?"

"Oh. Oh!" And he'd give a sort of hop-hop.

"That's good. Now can you jump with both feet at the same time?"

"Oh? Oh, oh, oh . . . ooh-ooh." And he would revert to his mannerism.

Luke seemed to have no knowledge of his body as a whole, and had trouble locating his body parts. He didn't always know where his head was; and if I asked him to touch his shoulders, he would touch his elbows. His concentration span was extremely limited, and any new movement I suggested seemed to trigger his mannerism. He couldn't manage a skip, but he would run a bit, and learned to slide. When I asked for a throwing motion, his hand would make a fist in the throw, and open up on the return. Luke cut off the air sharply when he inhaled, like a gasp, and could only release air in stingy amounts, keeping most of it stored up in his lungs. A tight tension prevailed over his body; he couldn't relax his muscles. He couldn't relax, period. He didn't know left from right, up from down, slow from fast. He wouldn't sit down or remove his shoes. He avoided being touched. And he wouldn't speak—except for his marvelous variety of "Oh, oh's." All of Luke's non-doings were performed with such a self-effacing charm that it almost seemed a pity to interfere with his behavior.

Luke appeared to be fascinated by his hands. He would stretch them out and look at them in amazement, then contort his face into violent grimaces of loathing. I tried to encourage him to make different movements with his hands, but he'd only fall immediately back into his mannerism. One day, I reached out my hands toward him in a gesture of acceptance and friendship. He stared at my open palms for a long moment, then uttered his first clear statement of fact:

"You are a white woman."

I think that some of the notes I made during the months that followed reveal Luke's basic conflicts, as well as the progress he made toward a more realistic version of life.*

. . . Luke always enters the room like someone who hasn't the right to come in. He steals in, as softly as a cat. But I think that his insecurity is tinged with curiosity. Today, there was the same preoccupation with his shoes. Once more, I asked him to sit down on the floor with me, and for the first time he made it. It was a very complicated maneuver, interrupted countless times by his getting up to rearrange the shoes to every point of the compass, and by frequent performances of his mannerism. But I feel that the ice has been broken. Luke speaks now, although very little.

*These notes have been abridged; for a more complete discussion of Luke see Schoop, Trudi and Mitchell, Peggy, *Won't You Join the Dance.*

He does take off his shoes. He will sit on the floor. His eyes follow me a bit more closely under their downcast lids.

. . . I told the nurses that I intended to enter his movement pattern. They strongly disapproved. He would think I was making fun of him. I might engender a "psychotic episode." He might never work with me again. Why would I jeopardize the contact I'd apparently formed? I went up to see Dr. Keermuschel.

"Go ahead, if you want to. It's an unusual experiment, but certainly worth a try."

. . . Today I decided to try touching again. Luke was in a good mood, and smiling a lot. First we touched our own body parts in time to a rhythm. When he touched his head, or shoulder, or knees, he doesn't give the picture of touching portions of himself; he looks as if he's touching strange objects. We worked with the beaters for a while, using them to touch each other's shoulders, elbows, knees. We stood up and did a few jumps and hops. Then I held out my hands to Luke and asked him to take them so we could dance together. He looked at them for quite a while, then looked away, muttering his "Oh, ohs"; then back went his gaze to my hands again. At last, very, very hesitantly, he reached out and touched my fingers—not really holding my hands, but sort of petting them in short, light tappings. He still made faces and twisted his body and peeked at me, but these reactions were less extreme than they had been the first time. We did a few more exercises. When the time was up, Luke made his usual farewell horns. I told him that in Switzerland, people usually greeted each other or said goodbye with a handshake, and I extended my hand. He took it. I gave his hand a firm clasp and released it. He whispered, "Merry Christmas," and departed.

. . . I still don't believe it! Luke came in very "normally." He said "Good morning" without the help of his horns. He removed his shoes and socks very naturally. He sat down opposite me and immediately went through his basic mannerism several times. Then he looked straight into my eyes, and asked matter-of-factly:

"Would you like to know what that means, Trudi?"

"I would like that very much," I replied.

"This," he said, demonstrating the bow and the horns with his index fingers extended, "is a salute to the white man. "This," and he made that same first movement, this time using the pinky fingers as horns, "is the greeting of the Boy Scout, or boy. This," the cutting gesture on the neck, "is wiping away the sweat, because I work so hard. And this," and he made the head stroking movement, "means that it's a hot day."

"Thank you Luke. Thank you very much."

It seemed that Luke had lifted a barrier that had long stood between us. We smiled at each other in mutual appreciation. I went on with the session, and it was a good one. In the past, Luke had frequently referred to himself as a zebra (black and white again?), so we went about on all fours, being zebras first, and then other animals. Luke enjoyed this play so much that he continued his four-footedness even when I wanted him to stand up with me and walk like people do. But I'm sure he was aware of the difference I was trying to make.

. . . "I went to school 'til I was five. I was a girl. Then I had a mom and dad. My dad bought a beautiful suit when I was eighteen or twenty; it had long trousers. When I went to church on Sunday, I had a dress on. I was a girl. Now I am . . . you know . . . sort of a man, or a boy."

"Could you show me, Luke, or act out for me, what you did and how you moved as a girl?"

"I held my left arm with my right hand. And I walked like this!" And he walked about, flouncing up and down.

"Luke, you are a man now. Show me how you walk today."

And Luke walked a masculine walk better than at any time before! Later, I tried communication movements with him. He did very well for a while, but when I asked him to show me in motions that he wanted me to come over to him, he didn't know what to do. He tried, but finally gave up the struggle, and just opened his hands helplessly.

. . . Luke had seemed to enjoy imitating people an animals, so today I began to pantomime different actions. I asked him to act out pouring some water, then drinking it.

"I get dizzy whenever I drink," he announced. "Even water makes me dizzy. So do all the liquids from trees. I even get dizzy when I eat."

"How do you walk when you're dizzy?"

"I walk just like I walked before!"

He insisted on this quite sternly. Then, after a slight pause, "I'm doing terrific. I mean, I'm doing very good. I'm doing okay. I am sixty now; sixty and forty is one hundred."

"You are forty now, Luke?" I asked.

"I was thirty-nine last year. I never was a baby. I was always alone—I had no father, no mother, no sister, no brother. I was all alone. Wouldn't it be nice to have a family and live in a town . . . you know what I mean?

We went back to pantomimes. I enacted looking around for something I'd lost, and asked him to guess what I was doing. His interpretation:

"You are looking to see if the janitor did a good job. You are a schoolteacher with a nice floor."

I did another one: I wake up in the morning, stretch, wash my hands, my face, my feet. Luke's interpretation:

"You must have a good time. You met nice people and you greeted them" (!!)

It was Luke's turn. He walked in a circle and made a deep bow. His explanation:

"I paced around on a big stage. It was thrilling."

When I asked him how he would wash his hands, he first plunged his arm downward, as if into deep water, and churned it around.

"I'm looking to see if there are snakes in the water." He washed his hands without rubbing them together. To wash his face, he ducked his head into the water; but he never touched his face. Then he said, as he performed the appropriate actions:

"Now I look up at the sky and see beautiful clouds—very white and hygienic. They come Sunday, then they disappear, then they come again . . . white, blue, pink . . . then they roll away." He made soft, rolling gestures as he crawled slowly around—as if he were moving through water. He looked up again and followed the clouds with his eyes:

"They come from the south, but they can't roll back to the south.". . .

Luke had another version of his fascinating past.

"I was a hyena . . . a milkcow . . . a beige dog—the head of a dog family—and now they say I am a human being. When I was a wolf, I met a sheep at the water. It gave me some water to drink. It was a young, beautiful sheep, about twenty-five years old . . . very friendly and nice. The wolf was exactly the same size I am. It was a big wolf.

"What happened then?"

"I made a rag doll. And then I made a grinding machine; and I ground myself . . . and the liquid became grapefruit juice . . . or, or, or . . . orange juice . . . oh, no, it was tomato juice.

When you put the rag doll into the juice, it comes alive. Any rag doll you pour juice over comes alive." There was a pause. "I had a sister. I wore dresses. My left leg is my sister's leg. The right is my own . . . chocolate and vanilla."

Luke certainly provides fantastic material. I asked him if he would like to act out the same scene with the wolf and the lamb.

"Oh, yes. I want some water. I have to protect my family."

I became a lamb, and Luke the wolf. I scooped up a handful of water and offered it to him. He knelt down in front of me and drank if blissfully. When his thirst was quenched, we jumped and leapt and ran about like two wolves. His movements and gestures were marvelous to watch. Finally, we lay flat on the floor on our stomachs and lapped water from the "lake." Then we changed parts and repeated the same actions, he as the lamb, and I as the wolf. After I had drunk from his hand, we hopped and skipped about like lambs, and again drank together. At last, we stood up, became erect, and walked together as "ourselves." And Luke's walk was amazingly different. His step was firm and secure. His body had straightened out. It was if he had clearly grasped the posture difference between an animal and a human.

. . . "First I was beige, then chocolate-brown, and now I am very dark," mused Luke this morning. "I was once a white man. And I think I will be white again . . . They say this is a hospital. I will be white again."

For the first time, I didn't connect his color fixation with his racial conflict. I felt that he was talking about well (white) and have been ill (dark).

The session began as usual. We worked on levels: exercising on the floor, taking sitting and kneeling positions, and finally standing and moving into space. Throughout the session, Luke was quiet, and more involved in what he was doing. As we parted for the day, he looked at me directly and said:

"I think I'm going to grow up now. It took me six months." We smiled at each other. He started out of the door.

Luke and I had been working together exactly six months!

Postscript to Dance Therapists

It is tremendously exciting to be on the ground-floor level of our ever-expanding, ever-changing profession. Not one of us knows today in what ways it will have grown twenty years from now. We can't forsee what new horizons will have opened up for us. For that reason alone we should experience as much and as many kinds of dance as are available today. There will be some new ones appearing tomorrow so let's get ready for them! And however we use dance in our practice, it must relate to our human quality. We must trust and abide by our humanity. For I believe that our "work" is our personal philosophy and our exciting vocation.

I sometimes wonder if we are not a little bit insecure about our young form of therapy . . . and that we therefore tend to lean too heavily on the well-established professions, letting ourselves be pressured into looking with their eyes on our treatment. We are young, but whatever we will find out—and I believe that we will find out plenty—will come from the power of dance itself. I feel we cannot rely too heavily on other theories. They can quickly become unyielding models. And dance defies the confinement of other disciplines.

I deeply wish that we all could have a humanistic education (besides that we should dance and dance and dance some more!). I feel that we should be exposed to philosophy and psychology, to all the arts, to science and technology. They all tell us about where we have been, where we are now, and indicate in what direction we are heading. They hold a mirror up to life; a mirror that reflects the million fold faces of mankind. They show us every nuance of Life's expression. With never-ending curiosity, they try to discover the meaning of existence. They ask and ask—knowing that there never will be a final answer. All these works are beautifully formulated fantasies and dreams. They are the vivid expression of man's soul.

Keep asking—keep dancing—and happy fantasies to you all!

Bibliography

Schoop, Trudi with Peggy Mitchell. *Won't You Join the Dance?* Palo Alto: Mayfield Publishing Co., 1974.

Chapter 5

C.G. JUNG AND DANCE THERAPY: TWO MAJOR PRINCIPLES*

*Mary Starks Whitehouse, DTR***

Genesis

Odd, but I turned into a dance therapist without realizing it, simply because no such thing existed when I started. In teaching dance, I was dimly aware of a different and new element. People would come up to me at the end of class and ask, "What *is* this?" They would go on to elaborate that when friends heard they were going to "dance class" they felt what we were doing was short-changed. When they tried an explanation of it, they found no accurate words. I would ask, "Well, what do *you* think it is—what do you get out of it?" The answer always had as much confusion as I had myself. It took a long time before our work together came to be accepted by us both as more, and less, than dance.

Please do realize that I am talking of the middle fifties. Dance therapy was unknown, much less named. One evening I was sitting in my living room—someone had sent me a medical journal containing pictures of Marian Chace doing work at St. Elizabeth's Hospital, Washington, D.C. I recognized that a dancer had made use of dance movement to reach people who had no intention of becoming dancers nor even of using dance purely as recreation. She had arrived at an understanding of what she was doing far ahead of my own. The fact that she was working in a hospital while I taught in a private studio deterred me not at all; I sent for reprints of her articles, eager to learn what she could say about her work. I found a point of view, a usage of dance that sounded familiar but unfamiliar.

Not surprisingly, the unfamiliarity existed in the places where her work was not like mine. No early experimenters could be said to be remotely alike. From the beginning it has seemed necessary to distinguish between therapists working in a hospital setting, therapists working under doctors in out-patient clinics, and especially, those working in studios. This chapter will be from the point of view of a teacher who worked largely in a studio. I started with dance as known material, going on to use it in ways, unsuspected before, that seemed to help people discover and deal with personal life problems. These people were functioning and what are called normal. Once I was kidded by Bella Lewitsky when she felt that the term "normal neurotics" was slightly funny. It is not slightly funny; unfortunately, people have just as many if not as flagrant problems as people in hospitals. It is only that they manage their lives with "quiet desperation," instead of being markedly cut-off from the rest of the world.

**Mary Whitehouse, DTR has a diploma from the Wigman School and studied with Graham. She has trained, and continues to train, professionals in California. She is completing her book, *The Moving Self.*

From time to time, other articles reached me. I began to be aware of others who thought dance might be useful in a new way. Trudi Schoop and Jeri Salkin, formerly teaching at Camarillo Hospital, announced private appointments for using dance as an "adjunctive therapy." Charlotte Selver brought her work in Sensory Awareness to the West Coast. Something was stirring.

At about that time, two major things happened to me. One, my personal life fell into shambles that ended up in divorce and left me with two small children to support. The other, I became a candidate for analysis with a personal patient of C.G. Jung.

I had the traditional modern dance training of that time—from lessons in "interpretive" dancing as a child to a diploma from the Mary Wigman Schule in Dresden, Germany. I had gone there because nothing in America allowed concentration on dance without falling into the category of physical education. I completely rejected basketball and tennis rackets as part of my preparation for teaching! The Wigman training prepared me for a particular approach although I did not know it at the time; it made room for improvisation, placing value on the creativity of the people moving. It assumed that you would not be learning to dance if you had nothing to say. After the Wigman School my education at home went on to include other teachers. I took Martha Graham's June courses for a good many years and went to Bennington Summer School of Dance before it moved to Connecticut College in New London. Through all of this I was, of course teaching as well as performing. Since I lived in Boston, the New England area opened itself up, pristine and unaccustomed to modern dance. Practitioners were already there but I arrived full of zeal, fresh, young, ready to convert everyone to the fact that if they danced they would feel better. How right I was!

Making a living had become doubly important because of the divorce and the responsibility for my two children; dance became a practical means of supporting us. In depth analysis I slowly gained a new understanding of myself and a different view of the world; it made me wonder if the old way and the new way must be combined. They could not run parallel, and I could not ignore one in favor of the other. Analysis does not put food in your mouth; it enables you to work in a characteristic outer way while you go on with this strange new inner work. My way was dance; yet I had to honor the new. The new would surely change the old.

Even without analysis, the break-up of my interest in dance had already begun. The fifties and early sixties saw a remarkably dull period. Early in the sixties John Martin, former dance critic of the New York Times, then at UCLA, remarked that modern dance was dead. I couldn't have agreed more. Without some kind of renewal, it seemed to me a sterile pursuit for further teaching. I hated the thought of going on with it year after year simply as a job—an injustice to it and to me.

Then analysis provided a different and larger *meaning.* Combining the artistic and the human meaning might bring together outside and inside; it might open the way I was to travel. Perhaps I even glimpsed that welding them together could result in a revitalization of what was now, at worst a trade, and at best a familiar but slightly boring art.

Looking back, my beginning is hardly recognizable. I over-simplified of course, seeing new concepts and meanings too easily in the movement of people I taught, forcing everything I saw into a preconceived framework. If I then fell back on what I already knew, remembered things I had already learned, I also stumbled on pieces of genuine experiment, moments of movement that allowed people to discover something different for and about themselves—not because I taught it to them but because I made an opening for that discovery. I began to find a place for myself.

Don't think that I was clear about my aims or even my approach; as a matter of fact I was clear only about the necessity. The reader needs to be aware that in talking about the middle fifties, the beginnings of a new kind of work, the pioneer is the most in the dark of all. A theoretical model was not thought of, was not being sought; at least, I was not looking for it. I was desperately trying to become clear as to what was going on—that would be enough. In the early days there were times after classes when many of us went out to coffee to sit for a long time, discussing—valuable discussions that revealed reactions and brought up questions. There were some questions I *could* answer, but more that I could *not* answer; they touched on issues I would have to face alone, as best I could. Often I went home wondering *what* I was doing and *why*.

Whatever it was, we were traveling away from dance. I had to call it movement. In order to find what it was that truly moved people, I needed to give up images in them and in myself of what it meant to dance. There was another possibility; to dance surely meant the making of a product, finishing a piece of work to show. I was finding more and more that the things happening in classes allowed pieces of movement, not dances; and that it would be more directly descriptive to call what the people were doing movement until such time as they themselves wanted to make a dance.

The word therapy was already creeping into dance language, from the medical and hospital model, I think. I had some resistance to it. It seemed to imply that I knew and that the person who came to me did not know; I had the feeling it could not possibly be true in my situation even if it was true of other people.

For me, a theory of what is now called dance therapy came out of years of doing, of learning by action and experiment rather than thinking, reading, or being taught by other people. It came out of taking seriously the questions and needs of people along with what they produced in me. I learned to let go when people did not like me or my approach, admitting hurt but going ahead. When the announcement came of the Schoop-Salkin "Adjunctive Therapy," or I received word of Charlotte Selver's weekends with Sensing, I had to overcome an initial insecurity that wanted to say, "Well, if they know what they are doing and they are doing it right, then I'm all wrong and might as well not be doing it." My present conviction that, "It takes all kinds," was not available.

I have to be honest—presenting a polished theoretical model to students interested in dance therapy, without admitting that it is achieved in the first place alone, with pain and struggle, may not be true for a second generation, but needs to be known. If it is not, such a theoretical model can be easily learned without any reference to personal gifts or temperament. It can be adopted wholesale and imposed on patients, as clearly as any teacher of dance takes an acquired style and imposes it on her students.

Theoretical Model

Can you believe how I resist the simple title, Theoretical Model? I associate it with an intellectual discipline, an organized rationality, that seems to me only one-half of a living process. Whatever theoretical model may be adopted, do not believe it is the whole. The whole can only be the whole *person*—to one teaching and the one moving in an atmosphere of mutual trust. A theoretical model that does not include this understanding is not complete.

For the sake of chapter space, I should like to emphasize lesser known, less understood aspects of my own theoretical model. My background with C.G. Jung leads to certain emphases as the main spring of my approach; I wish to dwell on these emphases.

Depth Analysis

When I refer to depth analysis I am referring to certain clinical psychological processes. The client/patient cooperates with the analyst to enter the unconscious, a realm below that of daily consciousness. This is done by using dreams, being particularly sensitive to images and their associations, becoming familiar with what Jung called *Active Imagination,* and generally accepting a symbolic understanding of life events, inner or outer. The process itself is one of discovering the living reality of the unconscious.

There are many kinds of therapy, many approaches to the entity we call the person; there are not so many approaches to a complete, a whole human being, including what is *not* known of the self down to a level belonging to human kind, not to the individual. This factor has occasioned the naming of Psychoanalysis and Analytical Psychology, as well as the Adlerian approach as *depth psychologies.* I shall emphasize particularly the relations between the two people in the studio for private sessions hoping these processes will be more clearly seen in an individual context.

"Self" and "self"

Because of the depth analysis I came to see and feel C.G. Jung's distinction between the many aspects of a human being, without his forgetting for a moment the wholeness of each one. It is a wholeness consisting of totality, completeness. Most people say, "self" using the small letter "s" to mean the ego, the individual, the personality. The world of the self is the world of the Me and all its concerns.

Jung says, "Self" with a capital "S" meaning also the world of the transpersonal, a world greater than the individual, more powerful than the ego. The Self is the totality of aliveness; it is wholeness, known and unknown, good and evil. If this idea lies at the bottom of dance teaching, then it becomes a primary value leading directly to another—that of self-knowledge. I use a wonderful quotation from Krishamurti who says, "Self-knowledge is not an end in itself; it is the opening wedge to the inexhaustible." Let me paraphrase. The little self becomes the one that struggles with self-knowledge, taking the familiar structure of the personality apart and putting it together again with new elements, new understanding; but the inexhaustible is the big Self, the Unknowable, God.

Individuation Process

The Self guides and directs the Me, once the process of becoming conscious starts. This is why a theoretical model must not be sided only in that which is reasonable. It must also include the irrational, illogical, unknown. Jung has said that the Self *will* make its experiment with each of us. The only real choice is whether we will be dragged by the hair or whether we will cooperate. Cooperation means the long journey toward what he calls Individuation—the unique and conscious development of potential in a particular person the slow unfolding of a wholeness already there. Through self-knowledge, individuation puts the ego in the service of the Self, the whole. The growth of personality is only possible through inter-penetration of consciousness with the unconscious.

To say it another way: the personality can be enlarged by understanding that a theoretical model has only rational, abstract or intellectual content. It needs also to be brightened, lifted, differently ordered by the penetration of the irrational and the instinctive—unexpected thoughts, unfamiliar behavior. If room is left for this second side, you cannot have a system of beliefs within which you safely function. If that is needed, then you can help people only to a certain extent and in a certain way.

Since people are functioning wholes, a large part will be unknown to you both at any point that you are together. Self-knowledge and an introduction to the inexhaustible are what people come for, no matter what they consciously name as, "the problem." They are people functioning as well as they can in their daily lives, but feeling a lack, something missing.

It is my experience that individual's cannot be genuinely themselves doing their thing without a good deal of probing (not always pleasant) into their motives and limitations. This is not introspection and should not be understood that way. Instead, it is introversion, the necessary looking within that our age has successfully escaped for the most part. Individuals are accustomed to looking outward, gaging reactions and responses by a set of conditioned and acquired beliefs. They are not accustomed to finding a world within that also conditions—influences whether its forces are recognized or not.

Polarity

How do these ideas apply to a theory of movement/dance? To apply them involves concepts uniting already known versions of dance use with what is unknown—the unknown assuming a new importance and weight. A primary one, *Polarity,* is present in the physical body, through the personality, into all the *pairs of opposites* including conscious and unconscious. Life is never either/or but always the paradox of both/and. This statement looks simple but it is not the way individuals live. Individuals live as if things were always a matter of either/or. They have but to choose and the opposite will go away. It is not true, is it? If you choose in life, you do not get rid of what you did not choose. There is no such thing as choosing only one end of the scale; the other end simply disappears from your awareness, exerting its heaviness, as in a seesaw, from below your consciousness. Black and white, day and night, masculine and feminine, are familiar pairs in our daily experience. In the world of movement a dancer does not stop to think of curved/straight, closed/open, narrow/wide, up/down, heavy/light—these are myriad paris.

Applied physically, it is astonishing that no action can be accomplished without the operation of two sets of muscles—one contracting and one extending. This is already the presence of polarity inherent in the pattern of movement. Most are not aware of it in this form, but it becomes recognizable in the act of walking. Normally, when there is no acquired distortion, the human being takes steps by opposing arms and legs, the right leg balances the left arm, the left leg opposes the right arm. Learning to change from the involuntary opposition of right and left to its conscious use is not at all easy, particularly in starting a forward motion. People have to see that they are freeing an arm and leg forward *at the same time* on opposite sides of the body. Once started, it is the powerful action of opposite weights on the two sides of the body that further lifts and carries us into the air. Leaps in a forward direction are a high, open extension of arm and leg against each other.

When the two complete sides of the body are opposed, left and right is learned—different but somehow mysteriously balancing. The opposites can balance but they do not always; sometimes one is more heavily weighted than the other. Left and right have many connotations. From the opposition of left arm to right leg to left and right sides. I remember I was struck by Martha Graham's description of the left as the "sinister" side of the body.

The left has its own special quality as related in Rumer Godden's book title, *The Left Hand is the Dreamer*. It is the left that is hidden, innocent, irrational, naive—there are many names. In contrast, the right stands for conscious, familiar, controlled, active. They are physical and psychological opposites.

An exercise comes back to me. I ask groups of people, sitting on the floor, to concentrate on the right arm—perhaps they can find movement with it by taking time with eyes closed. They can discover what sort of action the right arm is prepared to take, what movement it will make. Some people swing, some slash, some grab, some weave, snaking around their own bodies. This process increases in curiosity and intensity. To add, not to interrupt, I say softly, "Without pausing to think, simply choose the first word that comes into your head. Allow yourself to be stuck with that word; it is the name of the right arm. Let the arm go on moving and say the name silently; don't change either the movement or the word." This process is repeated with the left arm, taking long enough for a completely different experience—then choose a word, the name of the left arm. Afterwards I ask the people to put these two words together silently separating them by a hyphen, then to reflect on whether the two names represent qualities they already know or don't know of themselves. Sometimes individual people give examples of their discoveries. They tell aloud what a shock the names are, carrying as they seem to, a truth about themselves and their behavior. One man found that on his right, the word slash had occurred to him—on his left, the word swimming.

Often, the two sides are not discussed aloud. Instead, I ask that both arms move at once to see what happens to each quality (remembered and named beforehand). What now takes place is of the utmost interest to the mover. Sometimes, one arm wins over the other—the stronger over the weaker, of course, but also the less dominant, the one thought of as weaker can completely change the other. Rarely one are slightly influences the other and, both come to an entirely new quality that must be named something different. At last, the group talks.

This right—left polarity is a recurring motif for exploration in movement, just as up/down, open/closed seem to be. A girl who has danced all her life, but without this kind of awareness, was appalled to discover herself sitting on the floor with the right hand tightly grasping the left. As she turned her attention to this, the left hand doubled into a fist and tried to withdraw, but the right clutched tighter and tighter until the knuckles were white. During this time, she told me afterward, she was innerly screaming at the right, "Let go, let go!" It would not. Finally, the left twisted free, still clenched, the right still hovering claw-like, a few inches away. As soon as the left was free, she could no longer feel it though she knew it was there. She could only perceive the power drive of the right. Then after a series of experiments she was compelled to recognize, "But my left side will not do anything I tell it to."

Both these exercises bring us from simple recognition of physical opposites into a larger framework, that of self-knowledge, a sense that the opposites mean more to us, individually, than mere physical conditions with which to work. A dancer usually has a stronger leg; she balances more easily on one leg than the other or extends higher on one side. Dancers try to make the more limited side conform to the freer—they force the left foot to a point as hard as the right thereby running the risk of injury. This is totally unnecessary for non-dancers. It leads, as a matter of fact, to the either/or attitude again. It pre-supposes something wrong with having two different sides—but they exist and not only physically.

Authentic Movement

Polarity leads into other forms of the same principle. I discovered in working that movement, especially in improvisation, acquired of itself words to describe it. When the movement was simple and inevitable, not to be changed no matter how limited or partial, it became what I called *authentic;* it could be recognized as genuine, belonging to that person. Authentic was the only word I could think of that meant truth—truth of a kind unlearned but there to be seen at moments.

The opposite of authentic came to be *invisible.* When one is helping people develop all the natural functions and capacities of their bodies—when one is encouraging them to become familiar with themselves, one quickly runs into their lack of awareness in certain areas; they have thrown whole parts of themselves away. These are the invisible parts; no matter how much movement takes place there is a queer effect—it does not show in a genuine way, it is invisible. Not until these areas are brought into conscious belonging can their movement become authentic and the invisibility disappear. We are faced with a pair of opposites again—authentic as opposed to invisible.

In the same way, *"I move,* and *"I am moved,"* carry the same implication. Each is an act in itself, but a different act. "I move," is the clear knowledge that I, personally, am moving. I choose to move; I exert some demand (not effort) on my physical organism to produce movement. The opposite of this is the sudden and astonishing moment when "I am moved." Dancers are terribly familiar with, "I move"; they are accustomed to think they do it all, that they must exert will power and effort for each thing they want to have happen.

The moment when "I am moved" happens is astonishing both to dancers and to people who have no intention of becoming dancers. It is a moment when the ego gives up control, stops choosing, stops exerting demands, allowing the Self to take over moving the physical body as it will. It is a moment of unpremediated surrender that cannot be explained, repeated exactly, sought for or tried out. If it is used as raw material for a dance something is lost, but something has to be lost since that moment was an instant, a happening in and of itself; the structure needed for a lasting work of art is something else.

Once the mover has had the experience of being moved he knows it is possible; he knows he does not do it all. At any time without his choosing a sensation of being moved can happen to him. This is humbling and freeing for the personality that demands perfection, control, conformity—all the ills of our social training.

I am especially interested in the moment when movers, including dancers, find themselves moved. A girl sat cross-legged on the floor in the studio; she was a dancer of great facility. On this particular morning she bowed her head and closed her eyes, taking a long time to move. We put on slow rather innocuous music without a strong rhythm. Her head sank lower and lower—she leaned further and further to the right until she toppled over, spread out, and rolled at least a dozen times across the floor, all in one fluid movement. She sat up white faced and trembling with shock. Her description came, "I didn't know that would happen—I didn't do it." In this case, she meant I, the ego, did not assume control—did not produce the roll; her experience was of being moved.

Lastly, I want to describe the paradox in which the opposites are united; each becomes the other. This is the ideal—it is what is meant by both/and instead of either/or.

There is a saying that comes from Tao. It was not intended primarily for movement but it gives the whole of movement awareness a framework. "Non-action in action; action in non-action." Both pairs are in each half of the total saying. They cannot be opposed; they go together. For me it means that in not doing anything, something is done. In taking no action there is already some action going on. The other half indicates a parallel possibility. In acting, in choosing, there is no action—the Me, the ego does *not* do anything, does *not* choose.

Experienced in many moments, many ways, a balance between action and non-action allows individuals to live from a different awareness. They come to the place where they can view everything, from simple movement to the deepest and most poignant moments of their lives, with an element of detachment, having two qualities at the same time. It is not that they do not suffer, but that they know suffering is not the only thing; its opposite is also there. It is not that they do not enjoy; they know there is suffering. Finally, if they are lucky, they can contain, be aware of, both of these at once. Then something new is created; it is like the differing qualities of left and right; a third is found.

Active Imagination

I mentioned Active Imagination. It is C.G. Jung's term for a process in which, while consciousness looks on, participating but not directing, cooperating but not choosing, the unconscious is allowed to speak whatever and however it likes. Its language appears in the form of painted or verbal images that may change rapidly, biblical speech, poetry (even doggerel), sculpture and dance. There is no limit and no guarantee of consistency. Images, inner voices, move suddenly from one thing to another. The levels they come from are not always personal levels; a universal human connection with something much deeper than the personal ego is represented.

Moments of insight, brought into focus by Active Imagination, have a natural effect on everyday life. They reveal a direction and show a development, acting as support and encouragement for what must be lived through, creating energy for a next step. The use of Active Imagination in movement is peculiarly valuable. Every possible way I could devise to involve people in their own fantasies and images, even moving out their dreams, provide raw material for understanding themselves.

A young woman stood at the edge of the big studio space. In front of her there seemed to be marshes—water lay everywhere but there was enough dry land to pass through. She crouched, carefully putting one foot in front of the other, proceeding out into the space. The water seemed to come up around her; she felt as if it engulfed her and said to herself, "Oh, I must try to feel it, I must try to make friends with it." She sat down, allowing the water all around her body but not her head. No matter how she played, the head took no part, staying well out of the water. At last she felt, "no, no," the water was becoming deeper. She stood up and walked away.

The next week everything had stopped . . . all her images . . . even her material in therapy. She didn't know what to do. I suggested that we go back to the water and the marshes, and she answered, "You mean anything to do with water?" I nodded, so she went out on the floor and found water immediately. She lay flat this time, playing in it with her hands. It was very shallow, barely covering the ground and not going anywhere . . . again came the feeling of the head resistance . . . still she could not allow herself to put the head down. Suddenly she could not bear it; she got up and walked away. This time she found herself in a burning desert. There was nothing, absolutely nothing but the heat, no water anywhere—no people—nothing. You could see her body begin to claw, she said she was clawing in the sand to get at the water beneath the surface, longing to find it, somehow believing in its value now, despairing because it had disappeared. She couldn't get enough by digging for it; she couldn't get deep enough. It seemed cruel to leave her with that unfinished, incomplete experience, but we didn't disturb it. The refusal to allow her head, the thinking symbol to become contaminated with water, a symbol for the reality of the unconscious, had led to the stoppage of images (already few and far between with her), spontaneous material in therapy, producing a depression. Her discovery of the close connection between refusal to allow her head to touch even shallow water and the proximity of dry, hot desert with nothing in it was spectacular in its results. Perhaps she needed to live with the despair, feeling herself digging for the life-giving water.

One reason that the movement form of Active Imagination is so valuable is that it is extremely difficult to censor. One moves before one knows what is happening. One can stop oneself from writing words; one can prohibit certain pictures in painting more easily than one can stop certain movements that come out of preceding ones. One cannot pick and choose from spontaneous movement the way one can from drawings and writing. Movement, like dreams, is ephemeral, one cannot will to repeat it exactly. Spontaneous movement, rehearsed and repeated, loses the very thing it shows; that inner processes take physical form and can be seen, their meaning apprehended, their value received by the person out of whose body the movement comes.

A student in a workshop related, "Most important, though, was experiencing the way in which something long buried can be brought to the surface through movement; much less conscious than painting or writing it is doubly valuable. Until a conflict becomes manifest in some way nothing can be done with it; it will not paint itself or write itself. But the body moves constantly; it needs no tool, or time or place, it is always there, it needs only to be listened to. Presupposing a certain amount of honesty and desire for self-knowledge, it is the drum, the voice in the night that tells the hero where the battleground lies so that he may go forth and rescue the maiden. (Editorial note—some heroes are very sound sleepers and it might be necessary for a sprite to beat him on the head with the drum before he gets the message).

"So it is that an image wells up in the body and moves it in the same way an image springs up before the eyes and moves the heart (and again, the body, since there are often chemical and physical reactions to images—fear, trembling, sweating, blurred vision, accelerated heart beat . . . and if that's not the body I don't know what is). What I want to say is that *improvising is like active imagination,* that it cannot be done endlessly in a vacuum but it must in some way be brought to a more conscious level. What Mary is trying to do is to show a method of getting at human action within a framework of personal movement."

Role of Teacher/Leader/Mediator

Implementation of these central concepts of Polarity and Active Imagination depends on certain attitudes in the teacher/leader/mediator and the student/client/patient. I purposely put all three possible names for each person is present in the private session. Relationships of leading and following, whether in dance studios or in the hospital setting are as varied as the people concerned; but the necessary attitudes are permissiveness and allowance on both sides, acquired by practice. They cannot be present by talking, wanting or trying. The three names I have used already indicate three possibilities. One can *teach* something or *lead* something or be the *mediator* for something; all three happen at different times. The mover is sometimes a *student of movement*, a *client who comes for help*, or in the medical model, a *patient*.

A first and basic attitude of the teacher toward the mover is starting, (beginning) where the other person is. This sounds axiomatic; perhaps people will find it easier than I did. An analyst friend said to me, "Of course you start where the person is." I did not at all understand what she meant; I thought it a good idea if possible, but I could not see how it was done. My head was a jumble of preconceived notions, learned devices. I must have thought the mover was blank. Over the years, I came to see that this is the single most important contribution of the experience practitioner.

Starting where the client is can only mean willingness to be anonymous one's self in favor of observing, quickly and without barriers, what is available to that individual. When people first come, when we have been through whatever amenities we both feel necessary, I sometimes give an instantaneous choice for starting work. What would be most comfortable, easiest—lying, sitting, standing? The variety is amazing—some people lie, some sit and some stand, yet no two are alike. A starting point of this kind gives the client a chance to pick something of his own rather than being told to do a specific thing. Following what is picked, I find myself up against it since I then have to suggest the immediate next step—what to try. The queer part of it is that the client is both blank and innocent. However, there is a reaction no matter how small, whether verbal or non-verbal. The job of the teacher is to see how the one who is moving feels.

In order to go on from the beginning the teacher/leader has to be willing to use whatever she sees. It will be worthwhile to do successful things first; it allows the mover to find satisfaction in what is happening before strange or harder things are suggested. It is important that she not correct directly, but work indirectly to ask questions or make suggestions. She must never take away but always add something.

There are risks in doing it this way. One of the first is not knowing what will happen and being able to stand it; this applies to both teacher and client. A second is that long silences are necessary to provide waiting, a quietness into which the mover can sink, finding himself, then moving. Waiting too long can be as destructive as not waiting long enough. If, with experience, one gains a sense of difficulty in the mover, it is possible to break up the immobile waiting with a suggestion to help the struggle. This does not interrupt; it is an additional suggestion given by a quiet, disembodied voice that offers help.

As important as the basic attitude of starting, the teacher must be willing to give up all preconceptions, all ideas of what would be good for the person, all assumptions of the importance of what she knows. When it comes right down to it, *she doesn't know anything in this particular situation.* Therefore, she has to follow her hunches. Intuition is no longer a dirty word; some years ago it was. Perhaps one was afraid of it because it was so irrational and illogical—a kind of interrupting faculty, apt to disturb our scientific approach to life. It would not allow itself to be catalogued and place in a neat box.

Intiution tells one what to do and when to do it. In order to act on it, one has to be willing to make a mistake. The presence of what one calls a hunch in everyday language indicates a possibility that may or may not work. By acting on the things that come up within, by trusting, it is found that the more they are trusted, the more strongly they come. This gradually changes the work. It becomes not as logical a process but just as orderly; a different order than that of the controlling ego that grabs onto what it already knows saying, "I'll think it out. If this person can't do what I ask, then I must recommend the right thing next." It may not be at all the right thing. Perhaps one wants the person to stand; the truth may be that standing will not come, spontaneously, for weeks. The mediator must aks, "Why do *I* want the standing?" Another teacher's attitude might be called the willingness not to impose; to offer actions as suggestions. This carries an assumption that you may not be right or appropriate. I have known clients to pay no attention, to feel free to answer back or to vary a suggestion in a way I could not possibly have imagined. In the early stages I prefer to observe rather than to participate; the client can then become aware of beginning, of choosing. Since the process is a development of self-knowledge, the growth of individuation and conscious wholeness, there is no use in excessive verbal directions or explanations. Something being done will catch the attention forceably; and after it, one can afford to say, "Look, look: that was it. That's what you're looking for." It may be a little thing: a moment of genuine giving in, a sudden ease of movement. Whatever it may be, it is the expression of where the client is. There is nothing else to go by. A chance is taken when seen, a chance that has to be taken, or the development from that point cannot begin to be followed.

In turn, what attitudes does the client need for this journey formed by help from the observer and participation from the mover? The first discovery each can make is of the attitude already present: an expectation, a demand or a need may be uppermost. The psychological approach to the dance therapist could be one of assuming that she knows, that she doesn't know. It could be wanting specific answers to specific questions; or a feeling of having been sent, even a special sense of having come voluntarily, out of curiosity. The important moment comes when the client is what I call, caught. It is the moment when client and teacher recognize and accept the client's beginning attitude, *without judging it.* The cue is taken from you; the client is waiting to see what you will do or say to reactions presented. For instance, "Isn't that silly," is a common defensive reaction. If the dance therapist permits herself to be disturbed, to react by comforting saying, "It's not silly," if the observer does anything but perserve interest, sympathy and a waiting silence, the mover is apt to change to another attitude that might suit you better. This is not wanted. What is wanted is a genuine involvement; it is only from the involvement that the process itself can begin. Early interplay can come from the mover trying the observer out while she attempts to see whether she can get beneath barriers thrown to keep her from approaching. When the dance therapist does, the process starts; the client can be said to be, "in it," however superficially. Earmarks of being caught are various; one is the client's complete self-permission for openness to what happens. Usually a first obstacle is "monkey chatter" in the head, preventing the attention from settling into awareness of what is going on. Mental activity, voices that opiniate goodness, badness, grace or clumsiness, value or lack of value, go on unmercifully. The cessation of these opinions cannot be expected simply by request. The monkey chatter must be accepted as it is, allowed to proceed with as little attention paid as possible, until it becomes less and less important, disappearing when something has taken its place. Permission without resistance, without judgement, proves stronger.

Permission like this is a sort of allowance, but one can give permission to one's self, then allow nothing further. A kind of deadness results. It takes the form either of no further action or the dutiful development of suggestion with no real interest. The first attitude has not led to its second half; *allowing whatever happens to show,* surprising or unsurprising. This is difficult to talk about and impossible to generalize; everyone operates at a different level. Working with a dancer, or a dance teacher familiar with movement, presents entirely different problems than working with those who have never for a moment considered their own physical reality.

The allowance described permits the client gradually to take over responsibility, accepting to or rejecting suggestions of the teacher. I was working with a dancer and threw open the possibility of finding out what kind of day it was for her, not with words but in action. Why didn't she show it by moving rather than by telling me? Standing, she closed her eyes and dutifully waited to see what she would do; then she opened them saying, "I can't. It's the most unstructured, awful beginning that you could ask of me." We dropped it and moved on to another possibility. It is not necessary to analyze the whys and wherefores of the client's attitude. As a matter of fact, it gets in the way, fortifying and justifying resistance.

Permission to one's self, allowance of anything that happens, letting go; is the latter different? I think so. It does not mean what is usually called relaxation, a kind of collapsing, throwing away the energy to become limp, heavy, lethargic. It does mean mobilizing attention so that the energy can express itself. This attitude would be the *act of attention,* following what happens, concentrating on it. The movement leads and the mover follows.

Therapeutic Process

Does that make any sense? It is an unaccustomed way of working. The impulse to move, however, is something in and of itself. If allowed, then the observer and mover really do not know what comes next; they must follow in order to find out. The impulse may go on through various stages coming to a blank where it stops abruptly, or it may round itself out through an organic development to a natural ending. Such an ending must be recognized: the movement, this time, is finishing. Pushing it further would be padding. There has been no mental decision to structure or form it, to do it a certain way, to finish it. There has been only an authentic statement of followed intention—more simply, an authentic expression of the way it developed, and the way it ended.

The mistake of assuming that all improvisation has no form cannot be made. A great deal of it does not include form and is not meant for that purpose, but there comes a moment when the organic development of the movement problem takes on a form of its own—a natural form belonging to the movement itself. When I see it, I know that the movement has reached a level where the sticky, formless aspect of improvisation has been overcome. That in itself is a kind of progress. It should not, however, be desired before thoroughly indulging the other. As one psychologist said to me, "We are, after all, adolescents in this area."

Both people in the session can feel the moment when the movement becomes weighted on the side of the Self—of the new, not yet known. It is a moment telling both client and observer what is going on underneath. More is discovered than can be known by characteristics of time, dynamic, quality; more is found out than the conscious mind reveals. This happening is like a great iceberg: its tops may have shown all the time, a peak above water; one thought there would be more underneath. Then the iceberg tips over; the hugh underpinnings are exposed—the buried parts, the two-thirds that has been out of sight.

This is one of the great values of Jung's concepts applied to movement. The client needs to learn patiently and slowly that this is so; there is no selling it to him. It has to happen in the experience itself. The teacher also must be familiar with it in her own life. The truth of the irrational has already manifested itself to each, perhaps, in slips of the tongue (what we call in everyday slang, "Freudian slips") in dreams, in moments of uncharacteristic behavior, different than the person usually known.

Irrational truth is not a truth of the logical mind; it is a truth of the deeper layers. It offers renewing life energy stored in levels not normally contacted. The quantity of verbalization—how many questions, how much linkage to the personal life—is a matter for individual decision. The life giving quality of the irrational cannot be denied; slowly, a positive attitude toward it is built up. Intuition is a good name because it is an irrational function; it covers understandable concepts not possible to elaborate here. Suffice it to say that the irrational is the side away from the logical, away from the incisively differentiated thinking a client is more likely used to, simply because he lives in the kind of culture that he does. To let go the dominance of familiar functioning presents another form of the same attitude. Letting go is not only relaxing, it is giving up dearly held beliefs in favor of newly won convictions.

Setting and Structure

Eventually Movement-in-depth became the name of my approach. It took various forms. Primarily, I worked with a private practice consisting of individual hour-long sessions with men and women. There were groups but no longer classes; I gave up classes because I found I could not follow, closely enough, what happened to individuals.

When I began group work again, I started it as weekend workshops for men and women. As far as possible, I tried to have even numbers of men and women. Even numbers allowed separation of men into a group by themselves, leaving the women to work alone. It also allowed work in couples, a man and woman together. Since not all weekends could be balanced in numbers, I found that two women and a man, or two men and a woman, not to mention two men or two women together, was something else again. The problems of sexuality, the difficulties with touching and being touched, the fear of self-exposure, all presented themselves.

From 1966 on, I gave what I liked to call teacher-training workshops. It is unfortunate for this approach that I did not stop to think that real teacher training would mean a sequential and logical development from beginning to end of whatever time we had. Teachers taking training could have begun where I thought training began, going on to different aspects of movement and ending with some small sense of the completion of a process. Instead, they found that I was doing what interested me at the time. Often they received a natural impression; they, "know what Mary does." They would elaborate at home what I had been experimenting on with them.

I had not set out to train them as teachers; I only thought I had. I remember a June workshop when I was impressed that only teachers were enrolled. I tried to do what could respectably be called training. After a time, I thought, "Oh, to hell with it! I have to teach the way I usually do—reacting to what is needed and combining it with what I feel. We will make out of it whatever develops."

What I was really doing was exposing experienced teachers to a new point of view; more often than not, it involved a discovery of themselves—something not hitherto recognized. These discoveries had nothing to do with telling them how or what to teach. The fact that they took away from them any of the exercises, reforming and using then, was incidental.

Mostly, teacher's groups were composed only of women; only once did I have a single man. His comments are worth repeating. He was an experienced leader himself and, accompanied by his new wife, had enough courage not to be intimidated by finding himself in a strange group of women only. Half-way through we were talking one afternoon; he remarked that it was the first time he had ever felt completely outside a group, able to look at the woman's "thing." Apparently the atmosphere of women together is a different strong and tangible reality. Although he was accepted and, as he danced with single partners, could feel himself a man in relation to a woman, he remained outside the group. This demonstrated itself clearly when a number of the women took violent exception to his verbalizing the distinction; spontaneously, they surrounded him in a circle. The force of their movement brought him to his knees, then down to the floor. It looked as if the women were witches who had cast a spell over him, robbing him of power. He proved not to be helpless; however, with a mighty effort he pressed against the floor, brought himself to a crouch and slowly pushed himself to standing. Without touching the women, he moved to provide space and protection for himself.

Individual sessions and groups of any sort whether classes, weekends, longer workshops are very different. The atmosphere in each setting varies; energy provided by several people meeting together enormously buoys and supports the single individual. Once the fear of being looked at and any sense of comparison is overcome, interplay and interdependence can be a joy and a delight. In a group you experience moments having to do with the outer world: relations to other people, attitudes toward objects, feelings toward atmospheres or circumstances. The reasons people come to individual work include their particular relation to being looked at; some feel unready, even unable, to be group members. These people trust the teacher figure for more than they do multiple strangers. Conversely, there are people not ready to be looked at by the teacher alone; they want to hide in the group, feeling their anonymity less penetrated by "someone leading" if they are one of many. They, themselves, change the format when they are ready.

In private work something may be learned about one's personal relation to someone, but mostly what is discovered is not particular behavior within a group at that moment, but life behavior acquired over years, attitudes toward one's self *and* others plus whatever is lying in wait to appear, if allowed. Even the times that seem blocked and meaningless turnout to be real discoveries. In one particular session a dancer wanted to work with an object in the studio—a box that was square, rigid and unyielding. No matter how she tried she got nowhere; no life would start. She spent the whole session trying to find a working relationship to that box. Complete frustration was followed by giving up. In discussing it afterwards, she said without thinking, "It's just as damn unyielding and rigid and ungiving as my relation to R. . . ." This was a revelation to her. She had been dancing out the relationship without knowing it. Those same feelings in movement perfectly mirrored the agonies she constantly struggled with at that time.

The two forms of work, individual and group, have something in common. The top layers have to be distinguished before this commonality can be felt, but the underlying activity is an introduction to the reality of the unconscious, the other side of consciousness. This reality lives in each individual; it is the unknown balance of wholeness. It connects each person with the larger Self inhabiting everyone else and the surrounding world. The possibility of becoming deliberately acquainted with the known personality gives way to a discovery that something more needs recognition. The ego, center of consciousness, fights other patterns needing to be explored.

Each workshop contained a nearly equal number of technical exercises or actions plus improvisations based on group or single explorations of specific situations; images were given, pictorial beginnings, allowing members to find their own responses. A word of explanation about images, as they are not familiar to everyone. For example, I would tell them they were in a cocoon, asking whether it was large or small, whether it was stiff or stretchy, unyielding or movable. I asked also what they were going to do about being enclosed in it. This meant I called for no action other than whatever they found available. Another image had to do with lying flat on the floor, right hand imagined as being tied down, even growing roots into the ground; it could not separate from the earth in any way. (This could as well be the left hand or either foot; the difference is instructive.) They were to establish the feeling of an immovable hand, then explore their reactions to that condition. These are random samples of specific images.

In groups, people learned to encounter themselves and each other. Sometimes a workshop would lean more heavily on one activity than on another, either because I cared particularly about exploring it, or because their interest lead me. Once we sat in a circle; I asked them to become silently aware of the single person in the workshop whom they liked most and the single person whom they liked least. Then they were to draw lines (in their own minds) between themselves and the other two, making a triangle of a particular shape, depending on where each was sitting. Finally, they took turns standing up, calling the names of the others. Form where they stood, all three began to move in anyway possible. Perhaps an onlooker could guess who was the beloved and who the rejected from the way the movement took place.

Another time, sitting in a loose circle, each person had a chance to wander around inside the form. At length, there would be a stop beside or in front of one person. Everyone else watched the encounter between these two people. Sometimes rivalry and competition appeared, sometimes two like natures. There were distinct differences in relationship. At times one became weak, soft and helpless while the other nurturing and caring. We saw sisters and daughters emerge; we saw fathers and sons emerge. There was a surprising honesty of connection between the two people who chose to become involved. Most people moved from an exploration of the Me relating to an inner and outer world, to glimpses of larger truth, a transpersonal area where all are subject to a larger Self and the experience of wholeness.

Two endings, each discovered by the doing of it, illustrate what I mean. When it was appropriate, I lead the movers single file, gradually we joined hands making a chain that curved all over the studio. When the time came, I doubled back, closely facing the second person in line. We slowed down as we walked, each person rounded the corner, coming eye to eye with every other person in the workshop. It took some time but was immensely worth doing, stimulating consciousness in each of us, not only of those who were there, but of how we all seemed connected. When the last person had seen everyone else, a circle followed.

Many workshops end naturally in a circle, with or without the chain walk. We lift our hands together, palms closed in front of our breasts. In the language of certain religions this means, "The God in me greets the God in you." It is a statement for becoming aware again of our little personalities in contrast to the totality governing all of us.

Movement-in-depth, derived from my own experience of Jugian analysis, means—Physical Movement as a revelation of the Self.

Case Study

Since the movement history of a person is implied in the title, I am taking liberties with the plan. I cannot bring myself to think of this approach as a method which may be my great lack or it may be inherent in the approach itself. A primary characteristic, after all, is the unique dissimilarity of each teacher/therapist. The work has to become individually hers. Perhaps that keeps it from being a method. Examples are scattered through the text in places where I felt the material could not be understood without them. Perhaps this way of presenting a case study will further illustrate the values talked about.

The study is not of a person; it is of a process. It occurs to me to offer as complete a description as possible beginning with simple technical functioning including inner reactions that result from a given image connected with the physical preparation. This may allow more insight into my way of working. I intend to quote from various members of the same workshop, concerning the same piece of work. Memories of mine are not involved; these are actual records from the time.

The process concentrates on the same idea in several different ways. Physically, work begins on the floor, focusing quickly on the opposites involved in up/down. Each is explored specifically, definitively. Everyone then goes on to discover the movement possibilities of the continuum on which up and down exist as two ends of a single scale. This brings a pair of opposites into contact with each other. The third stage takes an image for, "The earth is my mother. The sky is my father."

P . . . wrote me a note, "The work had its greatest flash on Wednesday after we had started on the floor, feeling the contact of parts of our bodies touching, even pressing into and out of the floor. The floor became a partner; the focus was on the up and the down. Up and down became mutually inter-dependent; they connected pushing into and away from the earth; they connected lifting and reaching with sinking into the floor.

"For me, consciousness of extra meaning came when you developed the work already underway by saying, 'Now, the earth is my mother. The sky is my father.' It seemed so clear, pieces of difficulty I have experienced in feeling rootedness in the ground connected up my spine to the head in an erect posture. This has been something I have worked on ever since my first lab with you three years ago. I finally felt it growing through my spine, cat-like, onto my feet, even in standing and walking!"

"Those experiences came right into a sudden realization that I knew nothing of my father—up, the air and the sky; that I drew my own strength from the down—the earth, my mother to whom I have been very close. My father is unable to let his inner struggles out, to let others know his feeling. He is typically kind, gentle, and capable in many ways; but he works in an industry which frustrates and pressures him: television sound production. He has an alcoholic problem which I see as his means of coping or not coping with all of these things. What strikes me is the similarities I am now beginning to admit in myself to those I've known in my dance."

"What came to me was that all my dependency needs are down, maternal; until now I had not consciously faced the realization that a blank side of me, a missing part, a large hunk of the unknown lay in my not knowing my father, maybe not admitting my father in me at all. Down felt strong and solid. Up felt vague, indefinite, intangible, uncontactable. I was deeply moved to know that I needed the up, my father; and it (he) needs me too. I had been in tears the instant that you made the suggestion of the image. It seemed to be what I was already exploring without knowing why."

Three days later she re-read the letter, "As I re-read this letter it all still makes sense. I think there is significance in the fact that we had been working from a familiar point, 'contact with the floor' up to that which has been more difficult for me to sustain, a connection *inside* from earth to sky. Never having focused on the continuum as the connection between mother and father, it pushed me into the realm of my own personal, family background—difficulties and vacancies yet unacknowledged."

I have included this letter in some detail because it mentions the entire process much more clearly than the comments of others who picked out the parts most important to themselves. The familiar being on the floor through the development of an abstract up and down turned into an image of up/down, father/mother and brought this person into contact with her own immediate background.

Another member, E . . . wrote: "The up/down images left me comfortable on the ground searching above me into the sky, looking out through the side of my face, arms dead and powerless, hanging weightless. But then, 'the sky is my father' brought a hurt, a nausea of tears; for a father as untouchable as the sky who had hurt me, toward whom I could reach only a little always with fear of being hurt again. As I continue to work, it begins to fill the arms with strength, with a developing suddenly realized anger at his withdrawal. When the beating began, I glimpsed the power and extent of the anger—then it was over."

It is important to say here that up/down, sky/earth are linked with the principles of feminine/masculine that are, in turn, included in the experience of some people.

"Another day the masculine image came to be my father after several moments of no associations at all." She goes on to describe her personal father, and then says, "In writing about the father thing later, I realized how confused I am about it—him—it was full of discrepancies in father—Father. My own father seemed to have turned me over to God. My father was attempting to be that himself, a spiritual, ethereal man who never touched me, never felt about me at all as a human daughter. I felt I embarrassed him, he used to introduce me as his 'amazon.' So, I've been embarrassed about being that—as if people may be repulsed at the sight of me or I might upset them about themselves."

In this particular workshop we were emphasizing masculine/feminine, man/woman, up/down. In the beginning, they were all separate opposites; later they formed two ends of a scale. The picture of the earth as mother and the sky as father was an image calling forth any available responses.

B . . . writes, "When we worked again today, it was with stretching various approaches to being down on the floor with the earth as mother and the ceiling as father. I struggled with both, especially with the earth. I needed to get away from the earth, to go more to the sky but the sky was not strong enough to pull me up, and the earth holds on to me. I felt I had to take all that was available from both and find a way to reinforce, to integrate them in myself. I struggled to get up, even using the wall. At last I felt my own strength and knew I was standing on, above and below the earth but aware of the sky. I wanted to go further up and reach the father, but was ashamed with the mother there. This wasn't good enough, I needed to find more of my mother and father operating in me. This feels as if it needed support from the whole person in physical encounters, as well as in verbally expressing how I feel whether kind and positive or angry and negative. Slowly I am able to allow a little more, still with anxiety, the feeling that I am bad and wrong, that they will not like me. But each day puts another brick in the foundation, and I begin to feel sure, comfortable with what I am like out there in the world."

Now I come to a different form of the same thing; to me it is incredibly mysterious that each person, hearing the same image, can be affected so differently. M . . . writes, "I have to stay with the day that I cried. I don't remember ever crying like that, and I am not sure that I was finished when we stopped. I was not prepared for those words: 'the floor is your mother. The ceiling is your father.' I cried even harder when I tried to stand and realized I couldn't. The words I said as I went back down from trying and drove myself into a corner were, 'I can't stand it.' So the question is; what is it that I can't stand?"

These are all impressions of individual experiences, internalized by one person without reference to the other members of the group. I want to include one form of group encounter between actual men and actual women at a different time. In this chapter, I have given more weight to the private sessions; it is interesting that the quotes given have all, nevertheless, come from groups. Apparently, what goes on in groups can be individual; I do not think individual work can be group work. The kinds of questions, the kinds of talking that link it to the personal life are different in a private session and can be done on the spot. The quotes used are all in the form of personal letters written to me; they could only be individually followed up. I would not have known what the experience of beginning of the floor and following through the image occasioned in each person unless I had been told. In individual sessions, I would probably have been told.

The group encounter described next presents my point of view, from the outside, in dealing with an actual man/woman situation. It comes from a movement session held in Bethel, Maine for the National Training Laboratory, and is part of the general work being done by a particular group with a particular "trainer." I was the movement leader for all groups so I saw each person in the workshop every day.

This particular group had come to more of less a dead halt. Men and women were at each others throats; there was such a definite dislike that communication was stymied; nothing was happening. I was faced with this on the afternoon of a summer day without the least idea what to do. I record the actual happenings as best I can.

I took the break in relations seriously, to the point of asking the men to gather at one end of the big living room, leaving the women at the other end. I told the whole group that a closed wall shut them off from each other, separating the room into two halves. Within its own space, each group was free to do whatever felt natural; a long period of horse-play followed with many attempts at trying things, none serious or lengthy. Finally, something real began. At the men's end, some had gone off by themselves to exercise or simply to sit, reflectively, in corners. Two or three were engaged in playing games or persecuting each other: one fellow was forcibly dragged between two others to a satisfactory position and made to hold it. The five or six women were having an even harder job concentrating than the men. They were not satisfied until they got hold of several pillows they could throw at each other. This created a kind of game; they smiled and looked more pleased with themselves. They paid no attention to the imaginary wall; the pillow tossing yielded to approaching each other until they were all down on the floor in a circle, heads on the pillow toward the center, feet out, like little girls telling secrets.

It seemed to me that the two groups were ready for a recognition of someone else in the room. I announced softly that the wall had been lowered to shoulder height. It was now a fence that could be seen through. The men gave up their games, everything they were doing, and focused in the direction of the fence. Drawing nearer and nearer to it as they watched the women who paid no attention, continuing in their circle giggling and laughing, occasionally changing places. The circle had hardly any movement, but it did provide involvement—relationship among themselves if not toward the men.

After a few minutes, I encouraged the men to reach under the wire toward the women, making their presence known, asking for attention. One or two moved up to the borderline, reaching under and through, their hands spread out on the rug. The tension of their longing was obvious in their bodies, although they voiced no need nor any claim. By this time, the women had gotten to their knees or feet, slightly loosening and breaking the circle. One or two looked in the direction of the dividing line.

I remarked aloud that the fence had opened and the men could crawl through. At the same time I gave a soft warning, conveying that sudden movement, or an assault, might drive the women further away. The approach might need to be gentle, even tender. This provided an influence; their approach was slow, in most cases on the belly and the knees. The women, separated now, were lying or sitting all over their own space. One man led the way, giving the others courage. He crawled up beside one of the girls and sat for a while stroking her hair. Since there were not enough women to equal the number of men, some found themselves with a man at the head, another by the feet.

A freind of mine, an analyst, once said that a place exists where men and women do not communicate, cannot exchange their ideas or feelings. This group seemed to have reached that place. When they were put in physical touch with each other, the door opened and somehow the log jam moved, so slowly that it took many minutes. There followed a gradual growth of trust between men and women, between the sexes. They could accept each other again.

It was striking that the trust included getting to the feet; in some cases the woman swayed in the middle, facing a man, with another man behind her. In other cases, a woman and a man rocked together, arms around each other, or the man stood behind the woman while she leaned on him as they moved. There were many different ways of coming to a slow and reflective movement. It was impressive to look at, having, as it did, a quality of resolving something. I remember feeling humbled by my experience of now knowing ahead of time what to do or how to do it. For a long time I had no idea what would happen next. Eventually, it seemed to me that enough had taken place for then to go on; they could give up their defensiveness and begin work; they could communicate again. When the session was over, people stood around, talking more than usual, but also more slowly than usual. The man who had first led, detailed his experience of dancing with a man and a woman at the same time. This opened up other couples, other threesomes, to describe their own experiences. The whole group shared itself with itself. Gradually, one by one, they disappeared to find their trainer waiting in the hall. They approached him, faces more open than when they had begun. He breathed a sigh of relief; they all went into a room to work.

This is a different kind of group work than the other which yielded individual examples. It took place within the framework of Encounter groups (T—groups), and limited itself to the here and now situation. There is no hint of linking it to the personal life or to inner experiences outside the moment when the encounter was taking place. Yet, it presents the same kind of involvement and development in dealing with the man/woman opposition.

The reality of the opposites, polarity, is not limited to any familiar pair that can be thought of; it is a principle inherent in the way life is lived. What interests many now is how widely separated the function of men and women has become. Could the present attempt to equalize the sexes mean that the woman in the man and the man in the woman be liberated?

Bibliography

Brooks, Charles V.W. *Sensory Awareness.* New York: The Viking Press, 1974.

Durckheim, Karlfried, Hara. *The Vital Centre of Man.* New York: Fernhill, 1970. Distributed by Humanities Press, Inc., Atlantic Highland, N.J.

Frey-Rohn, Lilane. *From Freud to Jung.* New York: C.G. Jung Foundation, 1974.

Ghiselin, Brewster. *The Creative Process.* New York: New American Library, Mentor Pub, 1974.

Herrigel, Eugene. *Zen in the Art of Archery.* New York: Pantheon, 1953. New York: Randon Pub, 1970.

Jung, C.G. *Man and His Symbols.* New York: Dell Pub., 1968.

———. *The Undiscovered Self.* Boston: Little Brown & Co., 1957.

McGlashan, Alan. *The Savage and Beautiful Country.* Boston: Houghton Mifflin Co., 1967.

Progoff, Ira. *The Symbolic and the Real.* New York: Julian Press, Inc., 1963. New York: McGraw Pub., 1973.

Richards, M.C. *Centering in Pottery, Poetry and the Person.* Connecticut: Wesleyan University Press, 1969.

Sorell, Walter. *The Duality of Vision.* New York: The Bobbs-Merrill Co., OP.

van der Post, Laurens. *The Dark Eye in Africa.* Op.

Chapter 6

THE ADLERIAN APPROACH IN DANCE THERAPY*

*Liljan Espanek, MA, DTR***

Introduction

As I present this chapter an the Adlerian approach to dance therapy, it seems necessary to clarify some points. Although the basic philosophy guiding the process in therapy is Adlerian as I describe it, this can never be my exclusive consideration. It is best applicable with individual patients and in rehabilitation after hospitalization, for both individuals and groups.

With regard to the body technical approach, besides modern dance as a basis, many other views and techniques may be applied depending on the patient's situations. These approaches will be brought forward below. It is not possible to enumerate them here, I can only mention those physical techniques most often applicable which, when appropriate, support the basic modern dance and ballet training: relaxation techniques by Alexander and Jacobson; swing techniques by Bode and Medau (both of Germany); Dalcroze methods of Switzerland, used relating to rhythm; Yoga for the striving for inner peace; Dervish turns for trance; and psychodrama. Folk dance, gymnastics, and games are not frowned upon with the retarded or anything else for that matter which can reach the patient.

The process in therapy, if it remains alive, will, I dare say, often have the tight framework of a particular school of psychology. It is difficult to say where one ends and another begins. No doubt situations arise, where one or the other exponent has presented useful discoveries and channels of approach most perfectly suited for a particular case. One "borrows" then. The patient's improvement is the criterion.

This, I feel, must be stated as a foreward to emphasize flexibility and avoid dogma.

All the various techniques, and, in fact, all new methods appearing in the field of psychology today, are studied and if useful, applied and made a part of my work and training. I do feel that dance therapy must be eclectic to be fully effective.

It is this combination of the psychological with body techniques that I have called Psychomotor Therapy, de facto nothing but a more psychologically emphasized extension of dance on which it rests.

**Liljan Espenak is a fellow AAMD, and an Assistant Professor of Rehabilitative Medicine at the New York Medical College. She has lectured throughout the world on psychomotor therapy.

Genesis

It may seem strange to say about oneself that one was an Adlerian before one became an Adlerian. And, of course, it can only be understood to mean that the basic concepts of Adler's Individual Psychology corresponded to an amazing degree with the experience and subsequent theories formed during my many years of dancing and teaching creative dance.

My first encounter with the therapeutic process inherent in the dance, although unconscious, was during my training and performing in modern creative dance under Mary Wigman, at the time the most famous exponent of the new dance form in Europe. As she had worked in close personal contact with Rudolph von Laban, with whom she spent many summer workshops at the Italian Lakes, his influences could be clearly felt.

Laban was already then a great theoretician, someone the modern dance world was in great need. And Wigman, being extremely intelligent, was an ideal follower, as she contributed of her own creative talent to Laban's organization of space and dynamics. Unintentionally, this combination gave dance therapy its two most important facets; the free improvisation by the creative, emotional self; and the organizational structure needed to harness and project the emotions.

This gift was unintentional with regard to dance therapy. The purpose was pure art, the performance of dance. Only later was it possible to discover the real power of this dance art. First by experiencing the great changes happening in oneself and by observing those happening in the others, did it become apparent that personal development went hand in hand with artistic development.

Colin Martindale, (1975) writes about two kinds of thought processes:

> "The initial creative inspiration comes from a person's ability to regress to primary thought processes. The later elaboration requires the person to use secondary, logical thought to carry out the inspiration. Primary process thinking belongs to the realm of dreams and reveries, free association, fantasies and mystical trances. It is primary because it comes first in our mental development and is the basic stuff of the unconscious. In contrast, secondary process thinking is logical, analytic and reality oriented. Psychoanalyst Ernst Kris explains that creativity comes from what he calls, 'regression in the service of the ego.' "

The therapuetic effect of this creative process has been manifested by artists of all times, who withdraw within themselves during the process of creation, battling as it were with their "neurotic" conflict and emerging with their completed work; at that particular moment perhaps as balanced emotionally as they can ever be. In a small way this could explain the effectiveness of all the creative therapies.

I did not make a conscious decision to become a dance therapist. I was first a modern dancer and then became a creative dance teacher. In teaching how to create and perform, observation and experimentation continued. Somehow the teaching gained depth, and the learned experiences became useful as they were remembered and passes on. The power of imagination, of creating, improvisations became important messages from the deep unconscious or conscious mind, offering a new dimension to help form and structure (till then) unknown feelings. A moving inward, "In Search of Self," as Fromm calls it.

A part of Wigman's creativity training consisted of "exercises" in letting go of "thinking" to allow "feeling" to come to the fore. There was a clear distinction between "thought up" dances and emotionally experienced ones. I doubt whether Mary had ever studied or knew about the

Reticular Activating System (Martindale, 1975), or the newly discovered Alpha Waves (Brown, 1974), which when rightfully stimulated produce imaginative activities.

But the fact remains that before every concert, each participant had a moment of solitude and silence and a method of moving away form every day reality and thoughts into the world of imagination and their own art. Actors and almost all performers do the same. This contact with self could be discovered and developed as a technique to be a beginning of self knowledge and self improvement.

And so one could observe the psychological changes, occurring in students of longer standing when the physical development towards better functioning and harmony had gained time to become part of the personality. It became also observable that it was always the same personality traits which appeared parallel with the same particular physical problems, apparent in gait or posture. Over many years of consistent reoccurrences it became clear that these parallels could not always be coincidental.

Eventually a conclusion forced itself into the theories of teaching creative dancing (i.e., emotionally charged movements), a working theory based on the experience of the unity of body and mind. As part of a unit, any disturbance of the mind must affect the body, as can be seen in droopy heads and hesitant gaits, in withdrawn chests or pelvises. In reversal, as part of a unit, any changes occurring in the body must necessarily effect the mind of that body, and bring about parallel changes.

What had been merely a technical dance program for the improvement of the function of dance, paired with improvisations and dynamics of composition, gradually took on a deeper aspect. Definite use of specific body parts could touch upon definite emotional problems, sometimes eliminate inhibitions or fears, allowing for a freer artistic flow of expression in the dance.

It was at this point I felt psychological knowledge and training imperative.

From my Masters study in earlier years, I was not unfamiliar with the "three giants of psychology," Freud, Adler and Jung. Added to these were Reich and Wertheimer whose theories had made a lasting impression on me. From my body oriented standpoint it was obvious that Adler and Reich came closest to the usefulness in body approach: Reich because of his biologically emphasized approach to therapy, and Adler because of his complete wholeness of concept: body, emotion and mind embedded in the surrounding world. For this reason, I entered the Institute for Individual Psychology which offers a three-year course in applied Psychotherapy, and was subsequently trained in dealing with all the practical problems of neurosis, various techniques, schools of thought, and group dynamics, i.e., Adlerian Psychology as described in this chapter, and as applied concomitantly with the emotional physical therapeutic program.

During those years I created my own personal system of paralleling the emotional expressions of the dance with the psycho-dynamics of verbal psychotherapy, and found a startling abundance of descriptive words created by the close identity of mind and body. This has been of invaluable help especially in the psychotherapeutic approach to the retarded with whom I have worked for many years and who have to rely on their bodies for communication. Through the knowledge of this body-mind identity, specific emotions could be activated by stimulating the specific body parts, bypassing the disadvantaged brain function.

I found great support for our body approach in Alexander Lowen's Bioenergetic Institute, which at that time was in its earliest beginnings. *Physical Dynamics of Character Structure* was not yet published, but here were the ideas once learned from Wilhelm Reich, with whom I had once been invited to work. Lowen's modified theories were easier to agree to, and so I became a member, which I have remained until today, with enormous benefit. Here the theory of parallelism of body and mind conforms completely to the dance therapy principles, although dance therapy emphasizes body expressions and a structuring program more.

It is impossible for a thinking mind to embrace any concept 100%, to the exclusion of all others. There will be areas of divergence from the "orthodox" Adlerian techniques in this chapter, appearing in their related places. New methods and schools of thought have developed, and effective theories have been built on the new generation. It would be rigid not to be eclectic, but it demonstates the greatness of Adler to have built into his own theory the acceptance of timely changes. Every human is uniquely influenced by biological and environmental factors. It requires no effort of thinking to conclude that the uniqueness of individuals of today, with their entirely different environment, and to a great degree biologically stronger, healthier, taller bodies—must be different individuals from the populations of earlier periods. The body structure plays an important part in physical dynamics, i.e., dance therapy, new techniques and a new flexibility is required while still resting on the basic theories of Adler which take change itself into account.

One more thing could be mentioned here: Adler's simplicity of style. Directly and humanly, he explains the complexity of living for every patient to understand. He says: "Explain him to himself."

It is difficult to say, now, whether I have become a psychotherapist using the body as a tool, or whether I am a dance therpaist, using a verbal approach. While the length of this genesis may infer that my road was long, it has allowed for ample time to blend experience with the learning of theories. What developed has been called "psychomotor therapy."

Theoretical Model

It is strange that when writing about dance and psychomotor therapy the same thoughts and theories with the same semantic expressions occur, as when studying the theory of Alfred Adler. When glancing through his books, the eyes of dancers, are caught by such expressions as: contact, inner security, aggression drive, life pattern, imagination, degree of activity in mal-adjustment, expressive movements, sleep postures, creativity and goal orientation.

His field of psychological, human interest was wide and all embracing, but for the sake of this chapter, I shall endeavor to concentrate on the basic principles, the core of his psychotherapeutic concepts as applied in psychomotor therapy, and deal with them individually below. They are:

1. Aggression Drive
2. Social Feeling
3. Inferiority feelings (and Organ Inferiority)
4. Life style (Early Recollections, First Memory)

Adler's place in the world of Medicine began as a neurological physician in Vienna, Austria, which would account for his close consideration of the biological human as a great part of the psychological concept.

It is amazing to note how, so logically following his own theories of the individual's "life style," his earliest publication bears witness to his own basic life style and social interest as later presented in his theory of psychology. His first known paper (1898) was concerned with a public health problem which had as its purpose to better the health conditions of the industrial workers. He had already then developed a strong feeling of "social interest." His next paper was also related to social interest (1904), it was concerned with the upbringing of children, and emphasized the need to allow for the child's confidence in his own strength. "The child's self confidence, his personal courage, is his greatest fortune" (Adler, 1927). One should allow for the child's overcoming his inferiority feelings.

These two papers together with his theory of "Organ Inferiority and its Physical Compensation" (1907) were new ideas appearing in medicine at the turn of the century and thus introduced a new principle to clinical practice.

This, his first close linking of the organic functioning to that of the mind and emotion, and its interdependence, is the first premis for successfully using the body approach to influence the two other systems, as is done in dance therapy.

Physiologically it was always accepted that if, for example, one kidney was defective the other would compensate by becoming larger and more active, and so on with the other organs. Recognition that this compensation also occurred on the psychological plane and took part in creating neurosis, even relating the particular kind of neurosis to a particular organ, was Adler's great contribution.

His theory, therefore, naturally offers itself as a useful point of departure for comparing psychological thinking with bodily function and especially expressive movement, i.e., dance. Orthodox medicine may say that Adler departed from the accepted mode of research which, during this century, had to be done on corpses, rabbits, or mice. But science has up till now vainly tried to determine and crystallize the very essence of life: the movement, the change itself, growth. Perhaps one must first have accepted psychology as a direct parallel phenomenon of the organism, before one is willing to accept these psychology tests as being equally objective as the test results of blood pressure or heartbeat.

It seems that the new advances made in psychosomatic medicine during this century have supplied the medical field with another problematic discussion: the art therapies. What of the validity of treating emotional illness by focusing on the non-reasearchable elements of our being: our needs and responses to art, literature and religion? Of the arts the dance, movement of the body inspired by the emotions, would almost completely exemplify the Adlerian concept of treating the triune existence of the individual: (1) the *emotion* being the motivating force, (2) the *mind* organizing the action, and (3) the *body* performing it.

It is said that Adler did not agree with Freud on the theory of libido. It was understood at the time to refer only to sexual drives. However, this view has been modified by many later psychological schools, to represent the whole striving biological force itself, the life force, life energy, beginning with animal aggression drive and concluding with reproduction of the species.

In psychomotor treatment I embrace this last concept as an underlying dynamic principle. The work with the body in movement demonstrates constantly this original life energy, the animal aggression drives, as an original biological force, which, when absent, leaves the human being passive, lifeless and disinterested in living.

Paradoxically enough, Adler writes about this drive (which he does not call Libido).

> "From early childhood, we can say from the first day (first cry) we find a stand of the child towards the environment which cannot be called anything but hostile, one finds it determined by the difficulty of affording satisfaction for the organs. This circunstance . . . indicates a drive toward fighting for satisfaction which I shall call "aggression drive" (1927).

The Aggression Drive

The aggression drive is a very unsympathetic subject to most patients, seeking help for change and inner growth. And yet it is one of the most essential drives given to man or animal, when understood in its right meaning and context.

The colloquial use of aggression will describe someone taking away something from somebody or unrightfully pushing ahead of someone, imposing their person unwantedly or unreasonably. In order to do this a person must have aggression drive, true, but the choice of how to use it, and where, remains the decision of its owner.

When aggression drive is seen as our original life force, life energy, unconscious desire to live, it becomes an expression of health and natural dynamics, for which we must be deeply grateful, if illness or early repressions have not extinguished it. Dealing with suppressed aggression drive through dealing with anger is a frequent and important goal of psychomotor therapy.

By suppressing anger, the dynamic force inherent in individuals is simultaneously suppressed, "laid in chains" for all intents and purposes. Only in recognizing it can it be controlled and put to positive use. Permissiveness is a part of Adlerian treatment principles, although most therapists set boundaries for physical assault.

Without the biological aggressive drive and the pleasure principle, the inferiority feeling would not result in striving for superiority, but be accepted as unchangeable, as can be seen sometimes in the mentally retarded. Inferiority feelings then remain together with the developing recognition of the powerful surroundings, and acceptance of their interaction. The aggression drive, however, will lead to nonacceptance of this position and result in striving for superiority as means of obtaining the pleasure principle. Rowena and Heinz Ausbacher in the foreward to their excellent book on Adler's collected writings (1956), (perhaps the most authentic representation of his theories) do admit to the fact that many psychologists, both then and today minimize the differences between Freud and Adler, in this respect.

We find that in the striving to unify the body (first priority in the approach in psychomotor therapy which, in fact, *is* psychomotor therapy), must be accepted and dealt with. Adler's concept of the influence of organ inferiority and of his holistic treatment would point to this. The individual is body and a mind. He is first a baby (aggression drives) and then becomes a child (overcoming inferiority) and adult (develop social feeling). He lives in immediate surroundings, and first reacts to them. But he also lives in a larger social structure, family, neighbors, school, community, etc. As a result of the differences of these factors in its sum total, he becomes unique, his uniqueness must be dealt with in its entity, its wholeness. Therefore the emphasis on "Individual Pyschology" and the often used phrase: holistic approach.

Social Feeling

Individuals do not live in a vacuum. Society is all around us from infancy on. Interaction with society; beginning with parents, siblings, family, neighbors, community, school, work and our society at large—is unavoidable. If communication with any or all these factors breaks down, stability as a member belonging to the surrounding world, cannot be built, with the ensuing in securities, hostility, fears and anger.

Adler calls this relationship to the world the individual's Social Feeling. He considers the human as being socially embedded, from childhood on through adolescence to adulthood, and any failure to accept and cooperate with the world around him becomes crucial. Unwilling acceptance, therefore, is not enough, there has to be social interest available to prevent maladjustment. To Adler this social interest is an innate ability in everyone; rather, an original need—as one can learn from individuals who have been isolated by nature, profession or otherwise for any length of time, or punished by solitary confinement. Maladjustment occurs when this original drive remains undeveloped, becomes suppressed, or meets with frustration and disappointment.

This can easily happen in early life, by too strong competition perhaps, unreasonable restrictions imposed by the surroundings (later transferred to society), suppression of the individual's personal drives, and/or completely loveless responses. Instead of developing cooperative goals, the reactions become hostile and defiant; and the individual develops compensatory attitudes, a self centered goal of superiority-strivings, born of his feelings of powerlessness and inferiority.

Group dance in psychomotor therapy, especially dancing together, and interrelating singly with a group, is an ideal form for discovering and developing social feeling.

Group therapy has a relatively recent history. In Europe, Adler because of his interest in children, established guidance centers in the schools where he intertwined the children before a group of teachers and parents. They found, surprisingly enough, that the children functioned better before an audience, becoming more aware of their importance as well as realizing the adults genuine interest in them. It also impressed them that there were other problems like their own existing in other children, which made them feel less isolated and abnormal. These simple facts are the comon denominator in all group therapy from the simplest forms of dance therapy as given to the mentally retarded or severely mentally ill, to the most sophisticated verbal and creatively active forms, as in psychiatric verbal group therapy or psychomotor therapy.

The group is a safe place, where one can take more chances in moving out. It offers the possibility for giving as well as taking in relationships. It is accepting of ones suppressed feelings of fear and anger, it is supportive in breaking through isolation, it demonstrates ones own resistance and/or gradual changes as mirrored in the others.

The group dance setting offers the unparalleled opportunity to deal with all these feelings on a physical level. In group dancing the great variety of new movement patterns, to music or without, awakens and constantly renews the interest in the activity of motion in space with its new emotional experiences. There are moments of discoveries about oneself and others through encounters, moving parallel, circle formations with community feelings, group vibrations, progression on the three different levels (high, middle and low), and timing in interchange as well as all the imagery made available by the leader.

Some groups may concern themselves with expressing in movement dynamic subjects like "turning their back on each other and then facing," "sticking one's head out," "cohesion," or "leadership and dependency." There will be resistances, as always, which in this physical situation of visible movement becomes convincingly demonstrated, giving an opening for free discussion by the whole group. Being able to function successfully as a member of a group and fulfilling the demands put to him in this model of society, strengthens his ego and makes him more daring in similar situations in actual life. He learns to accept and understand differing personalities and the demands of consideration. Thus the fusion of Adlerian theory with dance therapy, creates a new combination of treatment: psychomotor therapy.

All groups will not be able to function on this intellectual level. Different methods must be used with other groups. One of the simplest approaches in leading groups is to unite the group through easy rhythmic movement, thus establishing a communal feeling at once as it is used in history all through the ages, as Sachs describe throughout his book (1952). The powerful force of rhythm becomes here the most significant factor for group feeling.

In a childrens' group again other methods can be applied. Imagery and fantasy, playfulness and uninhibited romping bring the truest reactions, and the fairy tales and unrealistic stories offer great possibilities for reaching their secret hopes or frustrations.

The methods are many, too many to enumerate, but the goal is the same. In all groups, the goal is social feeling, with the patient's ultimate return and absorbtion into society, capable of dealing with himself in relation to his surroundings: family, friends, work, community and the world.

Inferiority Feelings

The feeling of inferiority may well be one most easily responded to in psychomotor and dance therapy. Adler writes about the origin of this feeling.

> "One must remember that every child occupies an inferior position in life. Were it not for a certain quantum of social feeling on the part of his family, he would be incapable of independent existence. One realizes that the beginning of every life is fraught with a more or less deep feeling of inferiority when one sees the weakness and helplessness of every child.
>
> Sooner or later every child becomes conscious of his inability to cope single-handed with the challenges of existence. This feeling of inferiority is the driving force, the starting point from which every childish striving originates" (1927, p. 65).

Being dependent on parents, on all adults and needing to please to satisfy their needs, mold their different reactions to the world: to a punitive parent, a praising parent, a neglectful parent, or an uncontrolled unpredictable parent, all necessitate different methods of overcoming the children's dependency, and foster their drive for superiority. This may be quite overt, but more often unknown to the child or even later to the adult himself.

The unknown effect of these adjustments are varied. A strong child might "train himself" to disobedience, each time indivdually seeking to feed his "superiority" (his victory); another weaker child, may use the methods of obedience to earn praise and love. These same methods carry over in adulthood, and if social deprivation has added to the inferiority feelings, the reaction might well be an overcompensation of overcoming fear, that of aggression in its strongest forms, and even lead to criminality.

The deadly effects of the inferiority feelings can be imagined but also the great possibilities for successful treatment which dance therapy can offer. The fact that body and mind are one is recognized and the countless means the dance possesses for both stimulation and structuring the body can be experienced. It therefore, seems safe to conclude that developing the body, and giving it the basic security for its physical existence in the world, must necessarily have its feedback to the inferiority feelings, and as physical strength grows help remove it.

From the simple feeling of using the legs in bending and stretching to running and leaping, the recognition of physical strength creates a kinesthetic satisfaction, which is akin to strength. As the physical program continues and becomes more complex, the knowledge of one's inborn potentials and the building powers of training in every area, cannot but increase a feeling of self and all the new possibilities arising from it. When stamping around the room together with other people also stamping, expressing anger, revolt, or just a letting go of innate power, it cannot but result in a greater feeling of self, as a person alive. These are things patients have expressed frequently.

On the other hand those who have experienced a certain rigidity in themselves, inability to relax and join in with others in exuberance or exhiliration, can teach their bodies the physical letting go, floating on a swing or sinking to the floor. A great moment occurs when coordination in the development of "the wheel" (the coordination test, Espenak, 1971) begins to flow in a natural way, demonstrating the removal of an emotional block, till then interfacing with the natural function of the structure. From there the step to psychological insight is made easier. The recognition of striving for superiority, until then resented and suppressed, or expressed with all the ensuing negative reactions from the surroundings is also facilitated. When recognized and worked through this power is robbed of its great potential for harm and made available for positive use.

Where insight is not possible, as in the case of the mentally retarded, this physical approach becomes even more important. In the cases where intellectual analytical treatment is impossible, body analysis and directed stimulation of specific emotions through dance and dance exercises can lead the patients through a sort of structuring development of the psychotherapeutic process, working with the body-emotion feedback concept alone. This accounts for its widely accepted application in mental retardation.

Finding the Life Style and First Memory

While "the style of life" is the unconscious forming of personality originating in the goals of the individual, whether these be "useful" or mistaken," it becomes the therapist's task to help him change his outlook on life, to help him realize his own true potential and guide him to a positive application of his strength with more success in living.

The rationale of therapy would then be, that once the patient has discovered his mistaken goals, replacing them with new individually determimined ones, the new social interaction to his true self will help him discard the old ones.

Though simply summarized above, this is known to be a complex and painstaking process. On the other hand, the dance therapist feels that with the simultaneous approach of understanding the life style (i.e., the mental and the body—emotional) and the body "speaking" its own "language," two avenues of approach are available.

The body approach is a visible, demonstrable perception of self. It is difficult to deny, that the head is lowered, or that the chest is sunken, or that the arms are inactive, or in overcompensation that the chest and ribs are strutting forward, the chin protruding and teeth clenched.

With some experience, the therapist can soon make an hypothesis. Adler distinguished between hypothesis and general diagnosis, terming the verification of the hypothesis the Special Diagnosis. In psychomotor therapy a similar process of understanding the patient occurs, with the verification of the hypothesis through movement diagnosis tests. Ideally the special diagnosis concurs with the information obtained through movement.

To Adler the most reliable information of the personality was obtained by learning (1) earliest childhood recollections, and (2) dreams. There are other areas referring to the situational conditions which, although important, do not find their direct use in pyschomotor therapy (Ausbacher, 1956).

Adler explains the reasons for this selection, saying that there are no chance memories. Out of the incalculable number of impressions which meet an individual, he chooses to remember only those which he feels, however darkly, to have a bearing on his stiuation. The patient chooses, selects or even invents and distorts past events which are believed to be true. The resisting ones, who invent on purpose to "fool" the therapist are not considered here. (This information also has its importance.) In effect, it is not important in the final investigation whether the memory is true or not. It always reflects his inner life, and gives a clue as to the creation of the life style.

The earliest childhood recollections and especially the first memory (or what the patient considers the first memory) are often most "beautifully" portrayed in dance improvisations. It stands to reason that this cannot always be reexperienced in the first sessions. As with all the other movement diagnosis tests, the appropriate moment for cooperation must be sought. In some cases the poor body contact makes the inhibitory factor too strong. One may then wait and lay the groundwork for movement, or one may accept the patient's verbal description for the time being. In later approaching the experience in body terms, the emotional impact of the early trauma can be stupendous and may often lead to catharsis. Here too, ideally the special diagnosis concurs with the information obtained through the movement tests.

Amazingly enough Adler was aware of the parallel between mind and body already back in 1929, before anybody had mentioned body language or had any concept of it relating to psychological use recognized in medicine. Up to then body language was only in art, scuplture, or in the theatre, in acting, and, of course, in dancing. Non-verbal communication was silently enjoyed as a matter of unconscious manifestation of feelings, an actor's posture, gestures, gait, and the acting out of stories in ballets.

However, in 1929, Adler writes under the title "Expressive Movement and Attitudes:"

> "Let us first speak about the movement of the body. Everybody knows that we judge a person by his manner of standing, walking, moving, etc. Let us consider attitudes in standing for instance. We notice promptly whether a child or adult stands upright or whether he is crooked or bent. We have to watch especially for exaggerations. A person who stands too straight, causes us to suspect that he is using too much power to assume this posture. We can suppose that he feels much less great than he wants to appear. He wants to appear more courageous . . ." (pp. 58–59).

Here lies a beginning to our later research into the meaning of gestures and their use in the emotional interpretation of dynamics. Adler was even then already aware of the significance of a person's use of space as an indication of his life style:

> "We can see how all these things point the same way because every human being is a unity and reacts as such towards the questions of life. As an illustration let us take the case of a woman who came to a doctor for treatment. The doctor expected her to take a seat near him, but when she was offered the chair, she looked around and took a seat far away" (1969, pp. 60–61).

Nowadays this observation has become public usage. We have numerous books and theories on body language, which occasionally include spatial expression. It can, however, confidently be assumed that the scientific usage of spatial expression was the great contribution by the world of dance, where space is an integral part of the expression within the composition. The Adlerian dance therapist trained in the significance of spatial phenomenon has thus been confirmed in her use of space, as she has learned to psychologically apply spatial directions both for diagnostic purposes and for the general therapeutic treatment.

In the philosophy of medicine, true diagnosis, the thorough understanding of things present, also implies the right understanding of what has been and what will be, i.e., the change factor. Adler foresaw what later the dance and psychomotor therapist developed as a help in treatment: the recognition of movement, its change factor and the flow of the change itself, not merely the *poses* but the changes from past to present and future.

Thus Adler was inspirational for the development of the now constantly used Movement Diagnosis Tests describing the life style of a person in movement. It consists of a series of apparently simple tests, measuring the emotional state of a person on the basis of his movements, and the attitudes revealed through them. The description of these tests go beyond the format of this chapter, but they will be loosely dealt with in the Case History below (Espenak, 1970).

Role of Dance Therapist

Every relationship consists of interaction betwen two people, whether it be therapist-patient, teacher-student, employer-employee, parent-child, husband-wife, or just friends. In each case the interaction is different, as each person's personality, philosophy of life and station play an important part.

For the therapeutic relationship, between therapist and patient there exists many different views of what constitutes the most desirable and/or effective form for interaction. One is the authoritative one, perhaps closest to teacher-student; another is the love emphasized parent-child relationship, and then there is the therapists as a helping friend. These are the most frequently occurring ones, although there are many others in combinations. Perhaps Adler comes closest to the last one. In his view the therapist functions as a friend, fully accepting the patient's individual struggle for the realization of self, to which goal he, the therapist, has committed himself as a helper.

The neurotic or pathogenic person may not basically be so entirely different from the so called normal. As *homo sapiens,* everybody knows feelings of inferiority, frustrations, hostility, guilt and deep anger. How else could one understand a patient? But while one has learned, perhaps by more fortunate circumstances in early or later lives, or through personal efforts, to make the adjustments demanded by surroundings and life, the patient has lost out somewhere along the line on accepting society and its demands.

He has grown up in circumstances in which he has developed a way of meeting his fellows and life situations in an inadequate fashion. The role of a dance therapist, therefore, is to make systematized efforts to give the patient opportunities for new life experiences. He can help him make changes towards new ways of feeling and new methods of communication. It may be looked upon as "walking on new paths" with the therapist beside him.

From Freud on, all psychotherapists demand of themselves that they observe and listen objectively and non-judgementally but with great sympathy, and that they turn off all emotional and moral reactions while receiving the information from the patient. Freud even wrote once to Carl Jung that "psychoanalysis was at its innermost a cure through love." In one of his case histories he wrote that "liebevolle vertiefund," i.e., "loving asorption," was much better than "halbvornehme herablassung," "semigracious condescension."

I think that this has been the generally adopted belief all down psychotherapeutic history till today. Adler himself advocated this view and achieved great success especially with the emotionally disturbed children, whom he called "the troubled child" and treated with new and great permissiveness. He also talked about honesty towards the patient. One would say that this goes without saying, since it is closely paired with the responsibility of another person's existence in this world.

Taken for granted that professional knowledge must be of the highest standard and can never be considered completed, a therapist must have a deep knowledge of himself and his own experiential relationship to life itself and his fellow man, i.e., social feeling. The greater his experience, the greater his understanding of neurotic illness. The greater his knowledge of himself the easier his task of subduing any interfering subjectivity.

In practice no one has ever met an individual, familiar with his most primitive needs and with no unconscious conflicts. Thus it can leave no room for condescension in a therapist when dealing with other human's problems. Perhaps Freud was right: love is the greatest element in any helping profession, love—and then patience.

Case Study

Duration of treatment: 3 years

Sessions: One and a half hours weekly.

Identifying Data:

Nineteen year-old girl. Grew up in a small community, lower middle class. Parents both of recent European background, separated when patient was 13. Daughters lived with mother.

Father:

Had his own business, but later became a salesman. Subsequently married and moved to another state. There was seldom any contact with the father, although patient sometimes approached him for gifts of money for specific purposes. (Dependency need).

Mother:

Was a housewife, quite attractive, and after the divorce dated an older, well-to-do married man. She also frequently had other short-lived affairs, which her two daughters learned to accept without further questions, as a part of being female. (Later promiscuity).

Siblings:

One sister, a few years younger, very intelligent and always a "good girl." A constant object a jealously for the patient who always considered herself "a bad girl" (sibling rivalry). The sister had a way of dealing with her surroundings which (in patient's words) "somehow procured her the cooperation of the family." *She* could go to college. *She* could complete her B.S. in biology and zoology and was then working on her Master's while the patient had odd jobs of a menial nature. For the patient the constant failure to compete with this sister was a source of great inferiority and depressions.

History:

She and the mother were extremely close until she was about 17. Mother put her in charge (oldest sibling), possibly to relieve herself of time-consuming duties of motherhood; and when she acted up as a hypochondriac, she protected her against difficulties in school in order to use her at home. In fact, the impression they gave together was of two people having a secret between them, with the mother bestowing the girst of bribery for the wanted services.

At this time she started dating a boyfriend of whom her mother disapproved, violently maintaining that he had replaced her in the patient's affection and from then on her mother made life unbearable for her and there were daily fights. Whenever a young boy would get interested in her, her mother would ridicule him, and find faults with him, making the patient ashamed and doubt her ability to attract anybody worthwhile. This and her growing inferiority feelings made her think that she would have no success with boys and that they only wanted to use her.

Chief Complaint: (using patient's words)

Depression at failures in holding jobs, in getting an education, in improving her appearance were her chief complaints. She was obese (guilt feelings). She was unable to live alone, and to take care of her apartment and herself, as she completely lacked initiative (felt trapped). She could not stand up against strangers, gave in to almost any man and hatred herself for it (promiscuous).

She felt a need to re-adjust thinking and emotional processes and to change her life which was full of tension, insecurity and anxiety.

First Memory:

Age 2 years. Was in crib, mother left for the store, she felt "locked" in crib. She needed a bowel movement, but could not get out. She *felt guilty* but had to do the bowel movement in the crib and felt *dirty* and *trapped.*

Diagnosis and Recommendations: by Adlerian psychiatrist:

Character disorder. Passive dependency conflict. Psychotherapy was recommended.

Previous Treatment:

Before coming to dance or psychomotor therapy the patient had received verbal therapy for almost two years. The therapist had attempted to direct her interests towards becoming more skilled in her basic interest, art and the dance. After another failure, this time at attempting constructive learning by attending a summer school for dance; (but cutting classes and becoming a dropout) the therapist suggested an experimental series of individual sessions in dance therapy. Shortly after, the intensive treatments in dance therapy commenced.

First Session:

When patient came to her first dance therapy session she was a sloppily dressed hippie, dirty, stockingless, sandalled, in blue jeans, and an enormous poncho. She was exceedingly eager to dance, however, and selected some classical music to move to: Beethoven's Fifth Symphony.

Once started, she could hardly stop. Emotions poured out. She was indulging in her own feelings, as a person who talks incessantly. It was not possible to give significance to any specific one of this deluge of feelings as it showered forth. It proved, however, her enormous need for a cathartic outpour. There was no organization in the movements, no control or consciousness within the whole twenty minutes she danced.

During the following discussion which was more of a monologue, she showed a considerable amount of intelligence with a great discrepancy between *thinking* of the dancing and the *doing* itself. For the therapist it was a good hint about how the thoughts and intentions got lost on their way to the actual execution by the body.

Her body structure bore out the same disorganization, withdrawal of the pelvis, weak spinal column, lack of muscular strength and withdrawal of the head onto the shoulders.

Movement Diagnosis Tests:

After a few sessions, when the patient and the therapist had already made contact, the movement diagnosis tests could be made. These consist of a series of six basic movements, probing into the positive and negative components of the persons personality as demonstrated by his choice of movements, as well as his movement habits. They are revealed in the structure of his body and in his posture, they show how certain muscle groups have become over or underdeveloped, a shifting of body placement forward or to the back, depending on aggression (forward) or withdrawal (back) etc. The overall outcome of the movement test gave a picture of an aggressive, unbalanced, somewhat compulsive, but intelligent and quite gifted personality.

Test 1:

Demonstrated a weak *body image* by the failure to lift the body up on toes and to open the arms in a free open movement.

Test 2:

Improvisation to music revealed a compulsive need to express feelings with its profusion of gestures and indulgence of sentiment. It paralleled reports of the initial interview by the Alfred Adler Clinic: the patient's need to talk about herself and finding it difficult to terminate. But it also showed the wealth of creativity and aggression available, which could be constructively used.

Test 3:

Degree of dynamic drive: showed up clearly as being strong but ineffective. Weakness of the spine, mainly in the sacrum (from withdrawal) inhibited the coordinating flow of movement needed for the successful and full effect of physical effort. Such weakness will tend to give the owner a feeling of futility. In fact, in blocking the movements from the legs to the torso and vice versa, the disturbance in coordination has to affect all progression and other movement involving the whole body. The first aim of psychomotor therapy, would most often be to strengthen these areas, reinstate the right function in the body, facilitate and give joy in movement, and thereby change the feeling of inferiority and futility to one of accomplishment and power—in Adlerian terms, minimize the feelings of inferiority.

Test 4:

Control of dynamic drive demonstrates the ability to organize and move with control and purpose. But as the test before would indicate, the rating here was very low. Without coordination, control is difficult, and a great problem.

Test 5:

The weakness in the sacrum acted as an obstruction to *natural coordination—(the wheel),* resulting in an inability of the thighs to support the body strongly. (Compare feeling in crib: felt trapped. First unconsciously psychological, then physically, and then later consciously psychological and emotional.) This progression represents the most obvious example of the Adlerian concept of feelings of inferiority.

Test 6:

In the test for *physical courage or fear,* requiring a backward somersault, she was fearless.

Treatment

The following sessions were spent in dance improvisation giving her ample opportunity to release the feelings of insecurity, anger, fear, and disappointment. She danced and danced and then talked and talked about the memory material evoked. I empathetically shared her memories of her early years, the feelings she harbored, her competitive frustrated efforts with the sister, and the manipulations of her mother and sister, all relating to each other as well at to the momentary male in the house, acting as stepfather.

After each time she left with profuse bewilderness, excitement and over-enthusiastic remarks, but also with an apparent improvement in mood. For several months, she would endlessly emote, in accordance with her own choice. A good part of each session was given to a recognition of posture and proper walking, beginning with the animal walk on all fours. Although difficult to do because of the forced involvement of her special problem of her mispositioned sacrum, she showed an admirable perseverance and endurance with quick results.

The setting of limits was the first important step in the process of therapy. In the dance sessions this would mean that a specific theme was chosen for improviations to which we would adhere. It could be one of her own choosing, but once chosen, should not move into other surrounding areas. Knowing that her intelligence could be a good ally, the themes were chosen in the realm of images, such as king, power, and arrow, subjects which would encourage control, pride, purpose, and goal, and discourage released and free dynamics like the sea or fire. Each improvisation was followed by a "conversation" about the "artistic" deeper meanings of the images, the symbols.

Over a period of months we would also delve into the physical incorporation of these feelings, as we simultaneously body-technically worked on the weak body areas needed for these representations. Exercises and dance rhythms were given, effecting greater muscular strength (1) in the legs, "to stand your ground firmly," (2) in the back, "to counteract being spineless," (3) in the neck, "to hold your head high," "be upright," together with coordination exercises bent on the discovery of the movement sequences in the body, the flow. The patient's experience in dancing and artistic interest made these therapy sessions less painful than others and facilitated the therapeutic relationship. When unconscious resistances appeared some particular music was selected, giving rise to parallel or similar feelings and thus, brought to the surface, could be dealt with verbally.

The new and growing feeling of self took on various aspects. The newly discovered energy would look for outlets and jobs were attempted. When disorganization lost her jobs (library clerk, salesgirl, waitress) the frustration had to be dealt with. The jobs would last from 3 to 6 months, the longest time was 8 months. This was a minor victory.

During all this time her attendance to the sessions had been regular and her efforts genuine. Physically she had improved greatly in all the aforementioned areas, but the other, deeper problems had been revealed. As mentioned before, the sacrum, instead of being in a relaxed state, allowing the free swinging of the pelvis in normal progression, was tensely drawn inward creating a stong arch in the back, and throwing the pelvis girdle backwards in a retraction. This now became our second focus of attention. A program of relaxing the lower extremities was added to the setting of limits, while the session still offered ample opportunities for release of hostility with foot stamping and punching movements.

In this period during the release of aggression and its permissive acceptance by the therapist, the acting out of promiscuity became intensified and its efforts carried into the session, while emotionally swaying from rebellion to remorse to indifference. But highly motivated as she was by then, these stormy times were interspersed with positive new efforts. She subsequently applied to a university for further schooling and took responsibility for a job and apartment as well. Her work at school was satisfactory while her working habits became much more constant. After completion of her studies, she had saved money to go to Europe on her vacation. A great reward! By this time she was no longer sexually acting out. The feelings of being a worthwhile person had grown with her, and this became a positive reinforcement. She says about this time, however, that it was "a very lonesome period."

In the therapy session we now discussed and danced topics like "stillness," "out of a cave," and "conflict." Breathing became an all important issue with conscious realization of self through inhalation and exhaltation. The sessions were no more so stormy, nor was the verbal torrent as great as before. The emotions faced and recognized in the body as something of her own, something she could enjoy as a warm, human, living experience, or control if so needed, gave her a changed attitude toward herself and so a feeling of security. "I began feeling like a worthwhile person, I was productive, and I was accepted." All along the physical program continued, the improvisations and verbal discussions, changing the body aspects, successfully fighting obesity with exercises and realization of her love feelings (she lost 20 lbs.), improving the posture through and with the function of the legs. While the struggle has not ended forever, while certain elements of challenges still occur and the head and spine have not yet attained their final free uprightness, every subsequent session laid another stone to the building of her ego-strength.

After a year of what seemed constant struggling, began what appears to be a meaningful love relationship of mutual respect and hope for a future. In her own words: "now I have first begun to live." Through gaining her inner security the ground stones were laid for accepting the open need for the outside world, reaching out from her solitude to her fellow man. "Social feeling" had been discovered; and later, participation in my ongoing dance therapy group gave her ample occasion to give and take, and to test her new resources and inner security in interaction with peers.

In selecting this patient for the case study, from the many different cases in my private practice, my consideration was to most clearly demonstrate the application of Adler's psychology in its purest form, allowing for the parallel description of the dance and structuring programs as they went hand in hand.

And although it is far from my intention to foolishly intimate that all treatments run their course with similar relative ease and success, I am hoping to have shown what, in the area of neurotic illness, sometimes can be done through application of the joint approach of psyche and movement in dance and psychomotor therapy.

Bibliography

Adler, Alfred. *Understanding Human Nature*. New York: Greenberg Publishers, 1927.
———.*Problems of Neurosis*. Longdon: Kegan Paul, 1929.
———. *The Science of Living*. New York: Doubleday Anchor Books, 1969.
Ansbacher, H.L. and R.R. Ansbacher, Ed. *The Individaul Psychology of Alfred Adler*. New York: Basic Books, 1956.
Brown, Barbara. "New Mind, New Body," *Psychology Today*. August, 1974.
Espenak, Liljan. "Movement Diagnosis Tests and the Inherent Laws Governing their Use in Treatment," *The Individual Psychologist*. May, 1970, Vol VII, No. 1.
———. "New Non-Verbal Approach to Personality Evaluation." Presented at Conference-AAMD, New Hampshire, U.S.A., 1971.
Martindale, Colin. "What Makes Creative People Different," *Psychology Today*. July, 1975.
Sachs, Curt. *World History of Dance*. New York: Seven Arts Publishers, 1952.

Chapter 7

PSYCHOANALYTICALLY ORIENTED DANCE-MOVEMENT THERAPY—A TREATMENT APPROACH TO THE WHOLE PERSON

*Elaine V. Siegel, MA, DTR**

Genesis

The cumbersome name "psychoanalytically oriented dance-movement therapy" is an attempt by the writer to conceptualize a form of dance-movement therapy that addresses itself to the entire self not only the body of the person presenting him or herself for treatment. It is also an attempt to pull together the insights of dance therapy and ego psychology with the aim of making one single treatment tool out of these two separate disciplines.

While this is deemed impossible by the more orthodox members of both schools of therapy, clinical observation, successful completed treatments of many patients during ten years, and some research, point toward the emergence of a new treatment modality which, hopefully, will combine the best and most important theoretical and practical tools available to each.

Verbal interpretation by the therapist is an essential tool to help the patient span the gap between his or her nonverbal and verbal unconscious communication and his or her life experience. Conscious conceptualization of felt movement experiences is used to strengthen first the newly emerging body ego and body self, then the more mature, growing ego that, hopefully, can rely on trial action, or thought, before discharge of tension or reaction to stimulus. Interpretations should include references to transference, resistance, and life experience.

During many treatment hours and in many separate cases it become apparent that the beneficial effects of the dance-movement sessions remained unintegrated unless discussed in terms of the patient's life experience. The physical good feelings described by many patients following a dance therapy session can in themselves become a resistance toward progress if they are sought for again and again instead of being built into the treatment process as stepping stones toward organic growth. For instance, a patient who initially was frightened to breath deeply and regularly may finally overcome this resistance and be delighted with the elation or tranquility that are the results of egosyntonic respiratory patterns. If he does not understand what circumstance forced him into "holding his breath" in the first place, he will revert to his former mode at the first time of stress in his life. Restraining must be accompanied by insight, or, in the case of psychotics, by positive transferences to the therapist. Psychotics tend to see the therapist as a real object, whereas neurotics are always aware that the transference is an "as if" phenomenon.

*Elaine V. Siegel is a director and supervisor of interns at the Movement Therapy Department, Suffolk Child Development Center; she is in private practice; Ms. Siegel has authored numerous articles and is a lecturer at Adelphi University.

The implication of this statement is, of course, that the therapist is either working very closely with the primary therapist, or is herself equipped to make an entire treatment plan. In this contest catharsis is also seen as part of the treatment, not the goal. Catharsis, with its emphasis on the temporary absence of ego and conscious thought, can be either too frightening or addictive. One patient may never wish to lose his boundaries completely, as is necessary in catharsis, because he privately believes it to be a form of an annihilation and so leave therapy prematurely in fear; another may gleefully experience the same thing as a fantasized sexual reunion with the first oedipal love object and continue to demand more of the same without ever being truly gratified. Interpretation by the therapist based on improvisations and verbal free associations of the patient avoids both these pitfalls.

Abreaction is usually much more easily obtainable because it deals with relaxation of part of the muscular or other somatic defenses without the global impact of a catharsis. At the same time, gradual abreaction allows the ego to observe and integrate what was warded off before, so that psyche and soma can once more begin to function as parts of a whole being, instead of two separate halves.

The split between psyche and soma is an ever recurring, easily observed phenomenon in our society. An environment that stresses the value of reading skills in three year olds but fails to provide that same three year old with word concepts for his or her genitals and such basic concepts as "mad, sad and glad," readily fosters individuals who have to rely on rationalization and intellectualization alone to exist. The denial and suppression of inner body sensitivities and the inability to filter instinctual drives through a well developed, many faceted ego appears to produce either rigid, spiritually impoverished people or, on the opposite end of the developmental scale, individuals who are unable to make connections between their needs and their life styles.

More concretely put, one often finds parents buying toys that develop cognitive skills, or subscribing to programs that are said to teach pre-reading and reading skills through games and records, before they have toilet trained their child, or more accurately, have acquainted their child with his or her own body signals. Small wonder, then, when such a child learns early to disregard, or to view as insignificant, the messages of its own body!

Some of these children later rebel by overemphasizing the need to follow instinctual drives in puberty without regard for their own or other's physical boundaries. They become sexually and sensually promiscuous. They use their newly acquired physical genitality to search for the dimensions of body space, body boundary, rhythmicity, and all nonverbal forms of communication as though this would compensate for the lack of adequate total experience during their pregenital, preoedipal time of life. Others never become aware of their body-selves and pursue their barren lives with the sole aim of avoiding anxiety or stress.

It would be naive to assume, of course, that all splitting between psyche and soma is due to environmental influences only. Predispositions toward pathology are presumed to exist. Phyllis Greenacre speaks of a "predisposition toward anxiety," while Heinz Hartmann (1958) and Margaret Mahler (1968) postulate inborn weaknesses in the ego-apparati of those afflicted by the deepest psychic illnesses. Isidor Silverman (1957) developed a concept of egonuclei which he sees as staying immature and unsynthesized in the narcissistic disorders. Renee Spitz (1965) deals with the lopsided, or deviant, development that occurs when one or the other of the "organizers of the psyche," such as motility or speech, are not achieved at age specific levels. In other words, a whole body of theory and research exists that places equal weight to environment upon individual inner endowment, or lack of it, in the etiology of pathology.

All psychic pathology is seen by this writer as having somatic concomittants which often are viable and open to diagnosis through the particular form of motility exhibited by the patient. Muscular tension patterns, shallow or irregular respiration, arhythmicity in auditory responses, body-image distortion and restricted interpersonal nonverbal communications are regular accompaniments of all psychic illnesses. These somatic manifestations are often identifiable by their place in the developmental and maturational scale of life and thus give an important clue as to the true psychic age of a patient, or to where treatment should begin.

Conceptualizations as to symbolic meanings of body parts and visible tension patterns have been worked out by such clinicians as Paul Schilder (1950), Alexander Lowen (1967), Penny Bernstein (1972), Wilhelm Reich (1949) and others. Judith Kestenberg (1967) has contributed important work on body rhythms while this writer's previous publications have tried to pull together some manifestations of both normal and pathological motility with developmental stages (1970, 1973). However, the tempting notion of ascribing specificity to expressive movement behavior carries with it dangerous pitfalls. A shallow breathing pattern, for instance, may be the result of a traumatic life situation or a total inability to adapt to the demands of life, i.e., someone who as a child "held his breath" while mother and father were fighting constantly may now be a distrustful, anxious, and guilt ridden person who cannot breath deeply because this simple act might reactivate painful memories and require an entire reorientation of his thinking. Suppose after initially building a working alliance with the therapist, abreacting and reconstructing memories, the patient discovers that he had nothing to do with the parental fights, that he took all that guilt upon himself to maintain the fantasized perfection of his parents. Obviously, such a person is on a much higher developmental level despite shallow breathing patterns than a person who right at the beginning of life warded off maternal ministrations to such an extent that adaptation to the respiratory and other rhythms of the mother became impossible. The first type of difficulty discussed might result in a neurotic with a diagnosis of obsession compulsion while the second one would, of course, be autistic.

Similarly, a chronic childhood schizophrenic might walk about with locked knees because in his helter skelter, disorganized world his body image never matched sufficiently to include the conscious, useful knowledge of his knees while a neurotic may suffer the same paralyzing symptom because he has fallen ill of a conversion hysteria. One would be fixated at about 15 months of age or so, despite the fact that some of his other ego functions such as speech and intellect, might have gone on developing and thus present the therapist with the task of having to nurture an adult baby; while the other developed all the way to the oedipal phase, led a comparatively normal life and then, under the stress of real or imagined trauma, compromised with both id and reality in the form of his symptomology. Again, both sets of patients may have similar physical symptoms, both certainly settled for their particular pathologies because at the time this was the only response possible to them in that specific set of circumstances, but what a world of difference there is between them in the amount and quality of perception and cognition, and, above all, object-relationships!

If the dance therapist addresses herself with single minded devotion to the body self of the patient only, the initial beneficial impact is either dissipated or remains as an unintegrated, misunderstood lump in the patient's unconscious.

Theoretical Model

Psychoanalysis

In order to avoid misunderstandings, it might be relevant here to discuss the specific meanings of some of the terms used previously. For instance, it is common to hear someone describing themselves as "being in analysis." This might be a misnomer for a once-a-week supportive psychotherapy type of intervention and does not give a picture of the school of thought behind the treatment plan. Many variants of the Psychoanalysis developed by Sigmund Freud have arisen. For the purposes of this discussion, the original meaning of the word Psychoanalysis is employed. It is considered to be "a branch of science devoted to the study of human psychological functioning and behavior" by the American Psychoanalytic Association. As such, it is divided into three categories:

1. A method of investigation of the mind.
2. A systematized body of knowledge about human behavior.
3. A method of treatment of psychological or emotional illness.

As a therapeutic method, psychoanalysis encourages regression to the fixation point within the therapeutic sessions. This allows for the expression of repressed wishes, forbidden impulses and the recovery of traumatic memories. Through the verbal interpretations of the analyst, the patient can make new decisions about old, and usually erroneous, assumptions about his past, thus freeing bound psychic energy by resolving old conflicts. A minimum of three meetings per week is obligatory to keep sufficient energy focused on an orthodox analysis.

Movement Therapy

The word movement therapy is used here out of a need to define that area of motility employed by dance therapists which is not precisely dancing or improvising but does deal with body movement of a voluntary nature which can be influenced by the nonverbal and verbal actions of the dance therapist; i.e., having an autistic child sit between the therapist's legs so that they can open and close them in unison is not "dancing" but a preliminary step toward that goal. Breathing exercises with all patients are hardly dancing but profoundly influence body image and flow of motility. Thus "movement therapy" includes all forms of moving one might employ with any kind of a patient during a given session.

Ego

Ego was a word first used by Freud to define the total mental self of a person. In everyday usage, this meaning is still prevalent. For the therapist "ego" has come to mean that portion of the psychic structure which is influencable by the outside world and therapy. The concept "ego" is a construct which is seen as mediating between the demands of instinctual drives and outward reality. It is the buffer between the id and the superego. When it functions adequately, anxiety is at a minimum.

Body Ego

The body ego is the core of the ego, that part which is the first strutural entity to emerge out of the undifferentiated state present at birth. The body ego functions on the borderline of psyche and soma and is, in its primitive state, part of both. Developmentally, ego functioning is based on the model of body functioning. The body ego is also the receptor and executor of perceptions.

Body Image

A sound body ego is needed to establish an adequate body image. This is the mental representation of one's body at any given moment both a conscious and unconscious level. Since we laboriously establish our body images during the course of development and maturation, it maintains its fluidity and is influencable by both external and internal factors.

The body image is dependent upon the visual and tactile exploration of the surface of one's body as well as on the sensations derived from inner organs, skeleto-muscular systems and the skin.

Body Boundary

The body boundary is part of the body image. It depends on one's awareness of where one begins and ends. The melting into each other during orgasm is a temporary dissolution of the body image. During psychosis, many patients feel as though they had no beginning and end and experience inanimate objects as parts of themselves.

Body Space

Body space is another component of the body image. In this context, it is not so much seen as the kinesthetic, tactile, visual or auditory measurable and objective entity dealt with by experimental psychologists but as the felt, experienced knowledge of where one is comfortable in relationship to other beings and things. Some people need a little bit of space around to feel free, others need a whole room to know they are safe.

Id and Instinct

The ego in its totality is seen to rest on and grow out of the id which is the repository of all totally unconscious wishes and instinctual drives. The instinctual drives are the carriers of mobile energy and are present in their undifferentiated form at birth. Freud offered the following definition of instinct: "An instinct appears to us as a concept on the frontier between the mental and the somatic, as the psychical representative of the stimuli originating from within the organism and reaching the mind." The motivational force behind the instinct is assumed to be both psychological and biological. The two basic instinctual drives common to all are aggression and libido.

Object Relationships

Both these drives are essential if one is to form object relationships. Driven by hunger, an individual reaches out aggressively to mother who supplies food and with her loving care and libidinal availability tames the child's needs. As the ego's perceptions of this ubiquitous and ever-recurring cycle mature, so object relationships grow. Untamed aggression turns into useful energy as the real world is perceived as adequately need-gratifying.

Transference

In the treatment of all emotional and most physical dysfunctions, transferences of these early object relationships onto the therapist occur, as well as in all regular, everyday relationships. The resolution of the transference means the end of treatment since the old behavior patterns have been relived with a better solution this time around. Both positive and negative transferences occur regularly, just as one felt angry and/or loving toward one's original parents. A negative transference can be helpful in resolving old angry feelings but must be interpreted in or aid the patient in abreacting and resolving old conflicts.

Abreaction and Catharsis

Abreaction merely means to remove, to act-away-from. It does not have the same global connotations as catharsis when the whole being is swallowed by the letting-go. One may abreact, or let go, piece-meal, as in crying, or by tension release in specific body parts and still ask oneself "why." In abreaction, the observing part of the ego is still present while in catharsis it is flooded.

The need for abreaction or catharsis may occur when fixation has produced pathology. When too much stress occurs during a given developmental phase, growth is partially or completely interrupted and forces the individual to respond in primitive ways that are not in tune with the rest of his or her self. The stressful experiences are usually a combination of excessive satisfaction and excessive frustration and are hidden from the individual's memory by repression. Archaic ways of gratifying the self are retained until regression in therapy undoes the fixation and fosters growth.

Psychoanalytic Dance-movement Therapy

To reemphasize: the aim of psychoanalytically oriented dance-movement therapy is to provide an opportunity for the patient to heal the split between psyche and soma according to individual developmental levels. All the psychoanalytic concepts discussed above are used in conjunctions with movement and dance, mirroring and improvisation. Concretely, this means that psychotics need a highly structured, safe session in which positive transferences are encouraged through need gratification and body contact. The therapist might begin by simply mirroring, or if this is impossible, by encouraging exploration of directionality by placing her hand on her side and saying, "This is my side. Where is your side?" and waiting for the patient to respond. Often the response will be chaotic with an inability by the patient to find his side. Perhaps the concepts "touch" or "hand" will have to be explored first until the patient knows his body well enough to direct it consciously into space. When a session focuses on one body part, or one concept alone, it is a good idea to counteract such fragmentation by including some free dancing at the end, even if this is no more than an inept rock and roll imitation or swaying from side to side by the patient. Such activity at the end of detailed work encourages the awareness of the whole body.

With neurotics, the focus has to be much more on improvisation which is used as free association. Music selected by the patient might be a starting point, or the repetition and exaggeration of a preferred pattern of motility. When viewed from the standpoint of normal human development, a treatment modality that addresses itself to soma as well as to psyche, offers the advantage of paralleling, or imitating, nature's way of ensuring growth.

Human Development

Individuals are born with an undifferentiated matrix which obtains all of the future psychic structures in their immature forms. The sensorium too exists but also is immature at birth. As the neonate matures, so do his five senses and with them, perception, cognition and the ability to absorb memory traces. The initial total response to proprioceptive stimuli is given up in favor of partial conscious awareness of the neonate's own body as he responds to feeding, diapering, being held. Willie Hoffer (1949), in a classic paper, describes how the infant forms his first body ego through the integration of hand and mouth coordination during thumbsucking. This simple act of self gratification becomes the springboard toward further self-exploration. Hopefully these tentative steps are aided by the mother who furthers her baby's growth by giving him bright, soft objects to see and feel and who allows him to become aware of her own body rhythm by holding and cuddling him. All these early experiences, then, are entirely perceived through the body. Spitz (1965) speaks of perception as having the following components: Equilibrium, tension (muscular or otherwise), posture, temperature, vibration, skin and body contact, rhythm, tempo, duration, pitch, tone, resonance, clang, and probably a number of others of which the adult is hardly aware and which he certainly cannot verbalize. It is easy to see then, how the dance therapist with her emphasis on rhythmic activity and her attempts to elicit spontaneous movement can easily provide a corrective experience, even provide a renewed interest in time perception by merely allowing a motor activity to begin and end organically. This is true especially in psychosis where almost all experiences are somatized. Somatization is define by the American Psychoanalytic Association as the tendency to react to stimuli with physical rather than psychic manifestations. The infant reacts to painful stimuli with a host of somatic responses. With progressive maturation, somatic responses to stimuli are replaced by action and/or thought processes.

During normal development and maturation, de-somatization hopefully occurs so that immediate discharge action after stimulus is no longer required. In other words, one has learned to count to 10 before giving in to excitation or merely thinks, "I would like to kill that person" without actually doing it. Desomatization, then, is an absolutely essential developmental step that should not be confused with the blocking out of body feelings. It is the controllable quality of these body feelings and the ability to make use of them as guides toward harmonious, total living that marks what we, for want of a better term, call a healthy or normal person. Thinking, as well as feeling, is a trial action that ideally precedes true action.

Resomatization

Resomatization is a regressive phenomenon that takes place during psychosomatic illnesses and has its share in the formation of conversion symptoms. It occurs when the ego is so overwhelmed that it must regress to its former mode of expressing itself in somatic terms only, with total unawareness of the psychological causative factors involved. Actual physiological, often pathological changes takes place in the organs or body systems affected by resomatization although the actual psychophysiological mechanisms by which the mind effects the body have not yet been fully clarified. Examples of resomatization are: ulcerative colitis, asthma, essential hypertension and various skin disorders. Schilder (1950) speaks somewhat more generally on the unity of the body-mind and the interdependence of psychological and biological factors when he says that: "There is so close an interrelationship between the muscular sequence and the psyche attitude that not only does the psychic attitude connect up with muscular states, but also every sequence of tensions and relaxations provokes a specific attitude." Again, it becomes apparent that a dance therapist who is well trained can aid recovery by the offer of relaxing and strengthening exercises, eliciting creative free form dancing or otherwise addressing herself directly to the afflicted body-ego of the patient. The scope of dance therapy is indeed a wide one if applied in a psychoanalytically oriented frame of reference.

Patient Population

In psychoanalytically oriented dance-movement therapy, the patient is almost always seen on a one-to-one basis and never less than twice a week, often more. Group therapy is only recommended toward the end of treatment, or when institutional policies preclude individual work.

With all diagnostic categories except autism, regression toward the fixation point is encouraged in order to start rebuilding on a sound foundation. This means that after an apparent initial improvement, the patient may exhibit more infantile behavior for the time being. Hopefully, this can be confined to the treatment hour by interpretation, i.e., the patient should be made aware of the fact that memories and needs will make themselves heard that belong to the therapeutic relationship only and need not be acted upon in every day life. An example of this would be a lonely woman who previously dealt with her dependency needs by picking up men whom she then expected to hold her like a beloved child in exchange for permitting intercourse. During her treatment, she discovered that it was mothering she wanted, not sex. Anxiously, she thought herself homosexual when her need to be promiscuous disappeared and a warm affection for the therapist came to light. Dancing in unison with the therapist and asking to be held and putting her head into the therapist's lap eventually fulfilled this woman's expectations and provided her with enough object constancy to form a permanent relationship with a man. Since the diagnostic category involved was schizophrenia, body contact with the therapist as symbolic mother was freely used.

Deeply withdrawn individuals often become boisterous and aggressively hostile in the middle section of their therapeutic adventure, as though to make up for lost time, until at the end they settle into the mode of behavior specifically suited to themselves.

In this respect, psychoanalytically oriented dance-movement therapy is effective in the same way as psychotherapy in the lifting of repressions and recovery of forgotten trauma. However, in working directly through the body, memory traces often spring into consciousness more quickly than in conventional treatment approaches.

It is inappropriate to work toward catharsis or regression to the fixation point with autistic individuals because for them this would mean total disintegration and catatonia. In autism, there does not appear to be that original, sound foundation upon which to build anew which is regularly present in other disorders.

The Role of the Therapist

It is the task of the therapist to lend herself to the interpersonal relationship between herself and the patient in such a way that she becomes the screen that reflects the patient's fantasies back to her or him in a non-threatening manner so that old conflicts can become conscious and can be reexamined. Her own feelings about the patient known as countertransference, will alert her to inauthenticity of responses. Verbal and nonverbal interpretations ought to be geared to the patient's need, and the patient's need only, particularly during the crucial times when the patient is regressing and particularly vulnerable.

Case Study

The process of initial improvement, regression to the fixation point and eventual resolution of conflict was particularly clearly demonstrated during the treatment of a fourteen year old girl who came to the writer with a diagnosis by the school psychologist of paranoid schizophrenia but who, on closer observation, proved to be afflicted by a borderline personality organization. Otto Kernberg has characterized this particular type of pathology as analytically treatable despite a propensity toward temporary psychotic breaks. This kind of patient appears to function quite normally except in relationship to his or her particularly important objects. They become easily overwhelmed by the conscious needs and desires of their families and cannot separate their own demands from those of significant others. Important for the dance therapist is that Kernberg sees these patients as never having learned to experience their mothers as both good and bad. Their perceptions of one and the same person vascillate considerably. The wildly adored person of today becomes the madly hated person of tomorrow. With such a split in inner object representation, a split in the self-representation also occurs. The individual afflicted by a borderline personality organization often has difficulty in observing and correctly interpreting his or her own body signals and generally treats his or her own body image with the same lability as objects outside of himself.

Doreen's mother came alone for the first interview since Doreen herself refused to acknowledge that there might be anything amiss in her life. The mother, a frail woman who moved and sat with a peculiarly frozen quality, gave a long list of possible problems for her daughter. From being a top student with a superior I.Q., Doreen had slid into danger of being left back in school. She had totally withdrawn from both her family and her peers and preferred to spend her free time with her paternal grandmother who was the only one who could "handle" her. The mother experienced grandmother's ministrations to Doreen as an extension of a rivalry that she said had existed since the day she had married Doreen's father at age 17.

The family had recently imigrated to the U.S. from Central Europe and in some ways had found it difficult to assimilate, though the mother was proud of the fact that the father was a hard worker who had managed to provide his family with a home of their own. He was said to be a harsh disciplinarian who tried to force his three children into what appeared to him to be American ways. Doreen was the oldest, followed by a brother and a sister. As the oldest, mother reported her to have been her father's companion and plaything who was allowed to share his daily evening beer and was generally shown off to the extended family for her unusually good looks and precocious ways until the brother arrived and displaced Doreen in her father's affection at the age of four. Mother reported further that Doreen had strong temper tantrums ever since her brother's birth which in recent months had become even less manageable.

Toward the end of the interview, the mother signalled by an even more erect, frozen posture and wide open eyes that she had something else to tell me. Through experience, the writer has found that it is often effective to meet such an unspoken appeal by reclining comfortably in the chair, arms at the side, to leave the torso exposed and open with a slight inclination of the head toward the patient and a pleasant expression in order to show receptivity without urgency. As in other cases, this nonverbal response was met with alacrity. It was as though Doreen's mother had read and absorbed Schilder's statement that: "There is no psychic experience which is not reflected in the motility and in the vasomotor functions of the body." She told me that her husband habitually got drunk on weekends during which time they often had fist fights. In subsequent interviews, she was also able to admit that she found these beating sexually stimulating. Monthly interviews with both parents were instituted because suggestions to seek help for themselves were indignantly refused by both parents and experienced as hostility against them by the therapist. It was easy to see where Doreen's own denial of problems had its origin!

The father came only once. He had a halting walk, carried himself with bent shoulders folded forward and above a narrow, sunken chest and kept his eyes averted from the therapist. He spoke haltingly in broken English but was able to turn toward the therapist when she spoke to him in his native tongue. Despite his shrinking, almost cringing behavior, he made it clear that he was willing to "give therapy a year" since all his other educational measures, such as suspension of TV privileges, beatings and shouting matches between him and Doreen had failed. He also voiced his conviction that he was being "sucked dry" by his family's needs and that the therapist with her demands for payment was joining the list of people "out to get him." His view of the world as a personal adversary was closely paralleled by Doreen's conviction that teachers and peers were her enemies because they did not tolerate her day dreaming in school and on the playground.

Both parents conspicuously failed to mention three symptoms that helped to accentuate Doreen's isolation from her environment. All of which, fortunately, came to view at the start of therapy. A description of their discovery and disappearance follows.

The interviews with the parents had left grave doubts as to the suitability of treatment for Doreen in the therapist's mind because resistance to therapy by the parents seemed particularly strong and hardly open to resolution since they declined therapy for themselves. Doreen would have to overcome her own severe pathology while living in an environment that seemed designed to perpetuate it. How much could possibly be accomplished in the one short year in such a severe case? Typically, the parents had simply closed their ears and refused to listen when told that this was not enough time. They did agree, however, to three sessions per week initially for Doreen and monthly interviews for themselves, which subsequently only the mother kept. Doubts as to Doreen's accessibility were further reinforced after she herself was seen. She shuffled into the room with the defeated round shouldered walk of an old, disease ridden person. She barely lifted her feet off the ground but slid her feet along the floor as though to preserve her nerves from transmitting signals to awareness. Her arms were held closely and stiffly next to her body. Her torso was bent forward in an attempt to conceal even further her breasts that were already hidden under a loose, dirty sweatshirt. Her adbomen was thrust roundly against jeans and a coat that was several sizes too small for her while her large feet were stuck in a pair of brand new faddishly stylish shoes. The whole girl was surrounded by a particularly unpleasant, sharp odor. She immediately sat down and announced: "My mother wanted me to change but I didn't want to come here anyway, so I didn't."

"Perhaps you wanted to find out what was more important to me, your clothes or you yourself," was the therapist's response.

"I don't want to talk to no psychologist" came the gruff reply. At the same time Doreen pulled her knees up and placed her feet on a rung of her chair. Folding her arms over her chest, she made herself as small as possible. The therapist mirrored this and added: "I can make myself small, too." With a disgusted look, Doreen unfolded herself and proceeded to study the ceiling. "When you look at the ceiling you can make believe you cannot see me then you are not in the same room with me" was another tentative intervention, since it seemed more important to acknowledge Doreen's feelings than to correct her assumption that the therapist was a psychologist. Hopefully, she would soon feel safe enough to show more of her anger openly so that a more direct interpretation could be made. To the therapist it seemed that Doreen had folded herself into a ball in an effort to become inconspicuous and to present the smallest area possible for a retaliatory attack upon her hostile declaration that she did not wish to talk. Her response to the mirroring appeared positive despite its overt contempt. At least she had felt safe enough to uncurl into a more open, and thus more vulnerable, position while reaffirming her original statement. On a nonverbal basis she seemed to have acknowledged by sitting up that punishment would not rain upon her for voicing her opinion. The rest of the hour was spent in silence, with Doreen looking at the equipment in the room. Her eyes returned again and again to the drawing paper, pencils and crayons on the desk.

The first few weeks were thus spent in relative silence. Continued mirroring with simple verbal comments relevant to what was happening right then enabled Doreen to walk into the room in a less constrained way. Her anxiety lessened somewhat. She began to walk about and to explore the record player, records, toys and books. She closed each session by sitting in front of the therapist and looking hungrily into her eyes. This was permitted without comment or interpretation in order to give Doreen the certainty that all of her actions were acceptable to the therapist.

Despite Doreen's strange clothing and even stranger body odor, the therapist began to see Doreen in a positive light. Her attire seemed to serve specific defensive purposes, such as emphasizing her separateness from others. When one is not sure where one's body boundaries are, surely strong responses, and smells, might be indicated to delineate some individuation! Following this line of reasoning, the therapist felt that Doreen was asking for positive affirmation of her being by her continued staring but that the transference was not yet strong enough to bear the weight of an interpretation. Spitz describes the need of the young infant to see himself mirrored in his mother's eyes, and Doreen seemed indeed as helpless as an infant to deal with the realities of her life.

During the next monthly interview her mother confirmed the therapist's assumption. Doreen had become the laughing stock of her class and the butt of her teacher's ironic comments. The mother hastened to assure the therapist, however, that due to the expense of Doreen's treatment there would not be sufficient funds to buy more suitable clothing. Since the family had just purchased a new car, this was recognized as a destructive attempt at manipulation and interpreted as such. The mother corroborated with tears, renewed talks of fights between her and her husband and an urgent appeal to help Doreen.

Apparently the mother felt both guilty about her statements to the therapist and revealed that they had been recognized as a ploy because on her next visit Doreen announced: "My mother says I can tell you anything."

When asked what she would like to talk about, her answer was curt and to the point: "Nothing," she answered. Since her body stance at that moment did not look particularly defiant, the therapist felt it was time for some educative measures. Doreen listened with great interest when told that most people who came to see the therapist as she did either did exercises or danced with the therapist or in some way made use of the things in the room. Doreen made her first fairly long statement then and declared that she did not like exercises because they made her feel dumb, thought dancing mushy and stupid since that's what teenagers did, but that she might be willing to listen to music or to draw some pictures. Since she was unable to make a choice among the records in the room, she promised to bring one of her own next time and settled down to draw some pictures. Her first picture was that of a monster with a pregnant belly and a chain around his neck whose portrait was cut off in the middle. (see p. 100) "He looks as though he is suffering" ventured the therapist.

"It's not a he, it's a she and she's choking and angry," replied Doreen.

"I'm sorry she's so unhappy" ventured the therapist. "Why does she have such a large belly but no legs?"

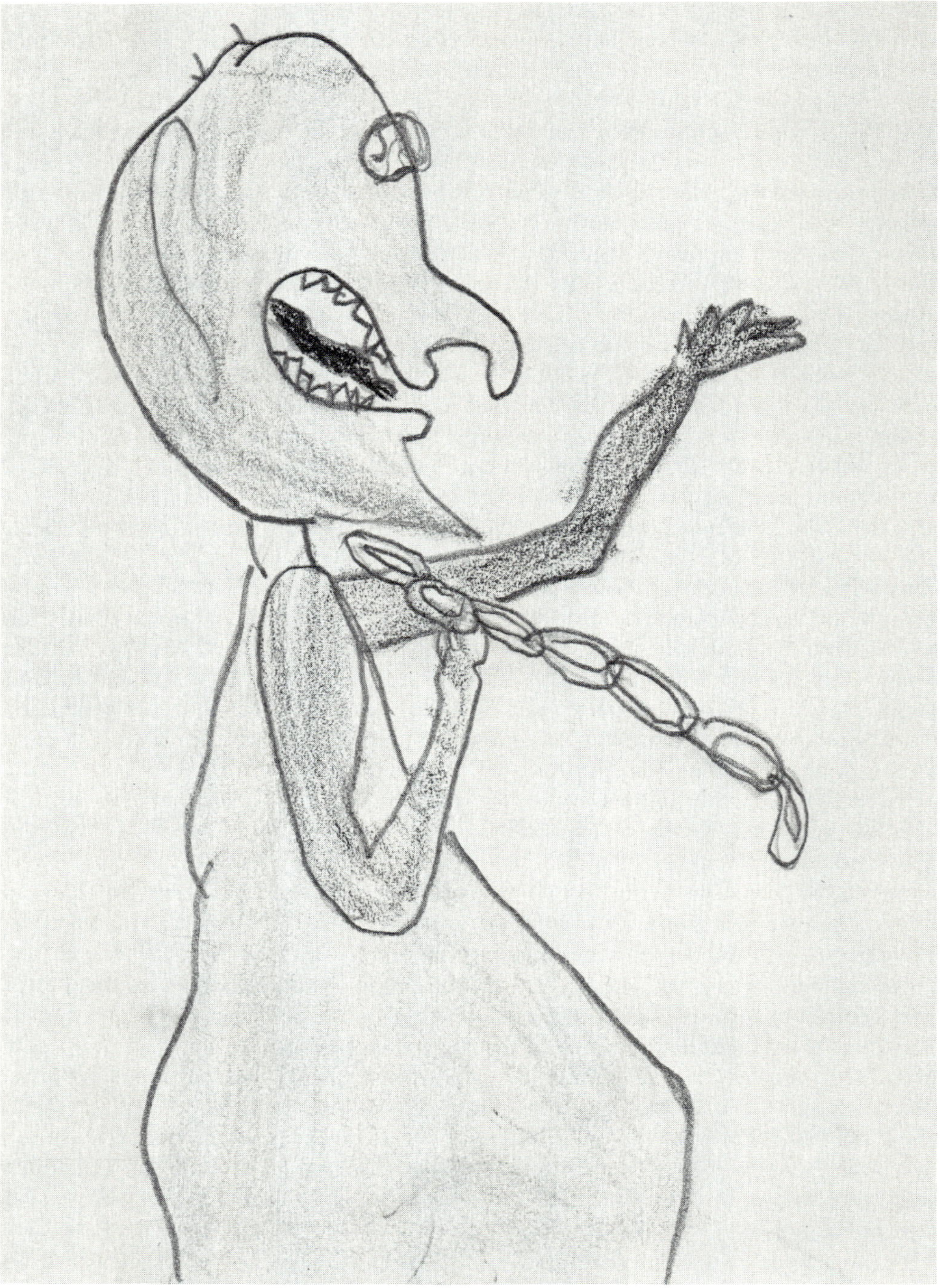

"Don't talk like that, don't you dare talk like that!" flashed Doreen suddenly. Her right knee had begun to bobble up and down uncontrollably. She tried desperately with both hands to hold it still, with little success. Noticing the direction of the therapist's eyes, she commanded, "Don't you dare look at that. It's none of your business. It's nothing."

Attempts at any form of therapeutic intervention were rejected furiously so that the therapist finally had to acquiesce in order to quiet the frantic child. It was as though joining Doreen in her denial of the tic enabled her to gain control of it. It was as though the therapist had to become part of Doreen's system of defenses. This was quite different from the symbiotic kind of union that occurs during the treatment of psychotics. During a symbiosis there simply is no awareness of the therapist as an other-than-I while during the enforced joining of Doreen's psychic structure, there was an awareness of the therapist as a separate being who must be controlled into sharing the same view of the world.

Because of this fleeting, if negative, awareness of the therapist as an other-than-I, it seemed plausible to assume that Doreen was not psychotic. Despite the incorporative aims of some of her behavior, such as the staring, there seemed to be some awareness of body boundaries and an ego that, though hardpressed, was still capable of rudimentary control.

Sensing the therapist's empathy, Doreen now began to talk volumes. In a flat monotone, she described rejection by her peers. She was fat, clumsy, ugly in their eyes. To prove just how clumsly, she demonstrated that she couldn't even skip properly and bounded across the floor with flattened vehemence to make her point. Finding the therapist unprepared to reinforce her body-image distortions, Doreen turned to tales of rejection by her teachers. They drove her to tears of frustration with their "meddling." Just what did she mean by "meddling"? For a moment Doreen hesitated and then confessed that the teachers would break into her favorite day dreams with their insistence on the boring classroom tasks at hand.

That Doreen's reality testing was severly impaired was clearly illustrated by the two examples above. Denial and splitting off of affect, as well as body image distortions were also present, as can be seen in the way she handled the tic and experienced her own motility. While her movements were heavy and bound, she certainly could skip and was far from ugly. The denial, or suppression of affect, was evidenced in her flat, dry voice that rolled quietly through the room with a quality of helplessness and hopelessness that quite belied the manifest content of her words. Her tightly constricted body stance and movements, the sagging of her shoulders, all pointed toward the painful storing of tension which hardly needed the irregularly erupting tic to underscore its existence.

When asked how she felt, Doreen was unable to describe any of the qualities enumerated above but drew, instead, a skeletal female holding her head. (See p. 102) Since the therapist guessed, correctly, that the pictured girl must have a headache, Doreen confessed that she often had them, especially in school. She was willing to do some relaxation exercises, such as sitting cross-legged on the floor and rotating first her head, then her torso and seemed delighted to "hand her heavy head" to the therapist. Gently holding Doreen's head and manipulating it until it felt loose, while supporting her forehead in the therapist's hands became a regular part of the sessions. Doreen was able to accept these ministrations because they were "like at a doctor's office. Not dance junk."

As her positive feelings for the therapist grew, Doreen finally kept her promise and brought in some records. They turned out to be "Claire de Lune" and "Liebesliederwaltzer," filched from

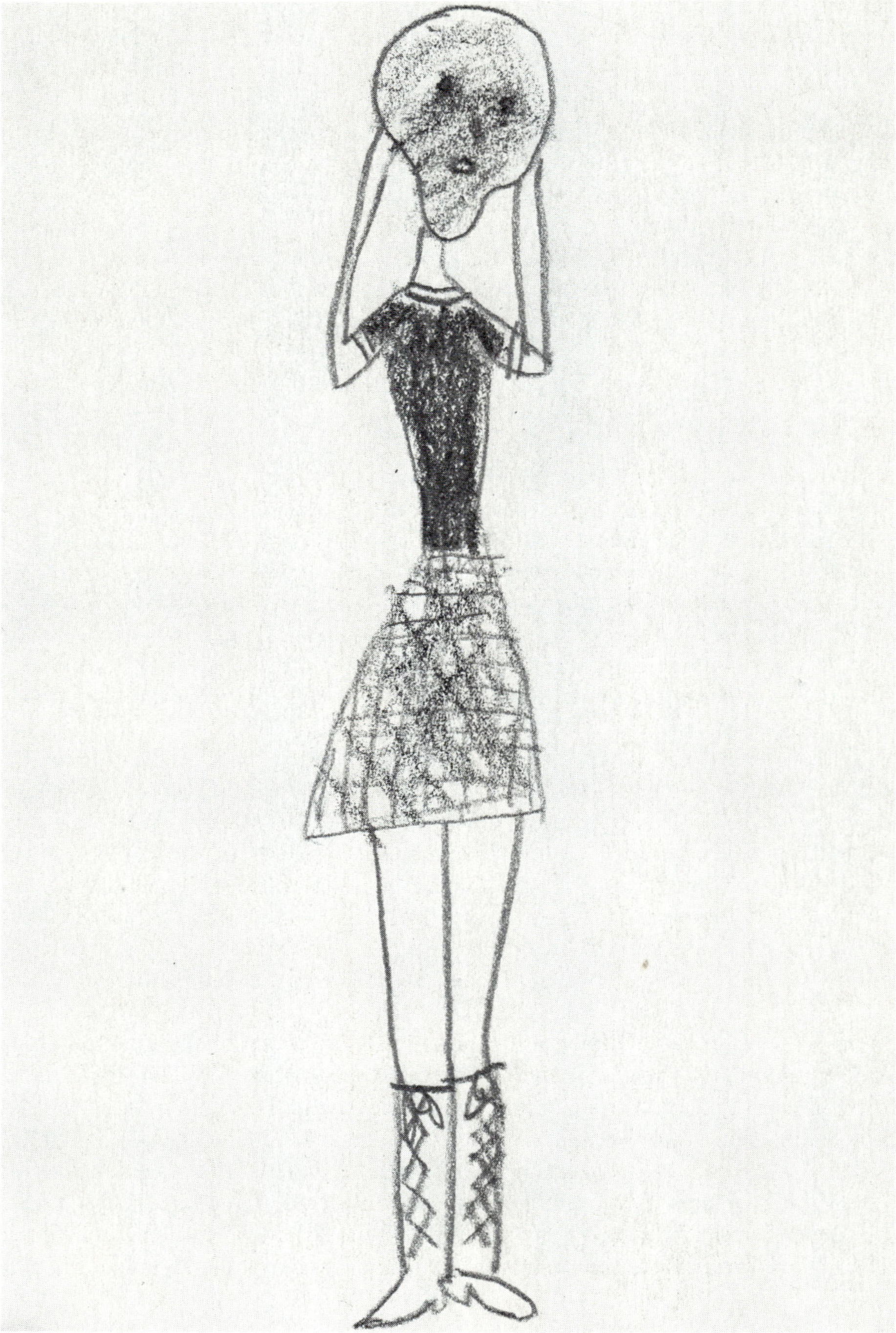

Grandmother where Doreen still spent every available free minute. Attempts to discuss why she liked these particular records and why she never wanted to spend time at home were simply ignored. Doreen continued whatever narration of rejection, to which a litany of people who gave her headaches were now added, as though no question had been posed at all.

Nevertheless, her mother mentioned that Doreen's report card had improved somewhat and that she no longer complained of headaches at home but had taken to fighting with her brother and sister in such a way that her father had sent her to Grandmother's to get rid of her. The mother seemed to understand that the father had reinforced Doreen's pathology by his behavior and asked him to mediate next time instead of "throwing her out." Doreen never directly mentioned this incident but assumed that the therapist knew all the details. The interpretation that the therapist was no magician, and had no supernatural powers and only knew what she was told, was met by an activation of the tic and an increase in fantasy production.

Doreen now began to talk about exploding monsters, monsters in the sky that hung there instead of stars and her own wish to be something else than human. During this time, an intense gender identity confusion occurred in which Doreen denied all knowledge of the physical differences between the sexes although she had participated in sex education classes in her school. She would tell the therapist about the fiery monsters; ugly, bloated, bodyless heads that swam in a liquid sky with hugh theatrical gestures and danced to a new record of her own choosing "In-a-Goddadaveda." Some affect had returned, but a totally inappropriate, not to say psychotic mode of expression accompanied her simple, though effective improvisations. Since none of her fantasy monsters ever had bodies and regularly exploded just at the end of each session, the therapist offered an interpretation that suggested the monsters as Doreen's own rejected, split-off negative feelings for her parents and her therapist who just hovered above her and then let her down and did not help her.

For the first time, Doreen acknowledged a verbal interpretation fully then. "Monsters don't go to the toilet" she answered cryptically but apparently following an internal logic of her own. The reply "but people do" had an amazing result. Doreen told of having suffered from noctural enuresis ever since she could remember. A device that was to wake her upon wetting had failed to train her, as had repeated spankings from both parents.

The symbolism behind the "explosions," however, was not only a need to suppress and express voiding simultaneously but was highly overdetermined. It stood in part for Doreen's headaches, her inability to control the tic in her thigh and leg, her displaced body feelings and her unacknowledged wish to know more about reproduction. All this came to view during the "working through" period after the initial revelation about the tic, the headaches, and the enuresis. While Doreen had acted in such a delusional fashion during her sessions, there had been some improvement in her school work and an attempt to make her nuclear family more aware of her. But once all the fantasy material had been presented to the therapist, an infantilization took place that nearly curtailed Doreen's treatment. She simply declined to speak to her parents at all. She also fell silent in her sessions but began to hop, skip and jump with glee every time she came. Sometimes, she would draw highly abstract designs that seemed to mirror her regression in terms of disintegrating body image but revealed a high degree of intelligence, creativity and organizational ability. (See p. 104–106) Her parents threatened to remove her from treatment and were persuaded with difficulty to endure this regression.

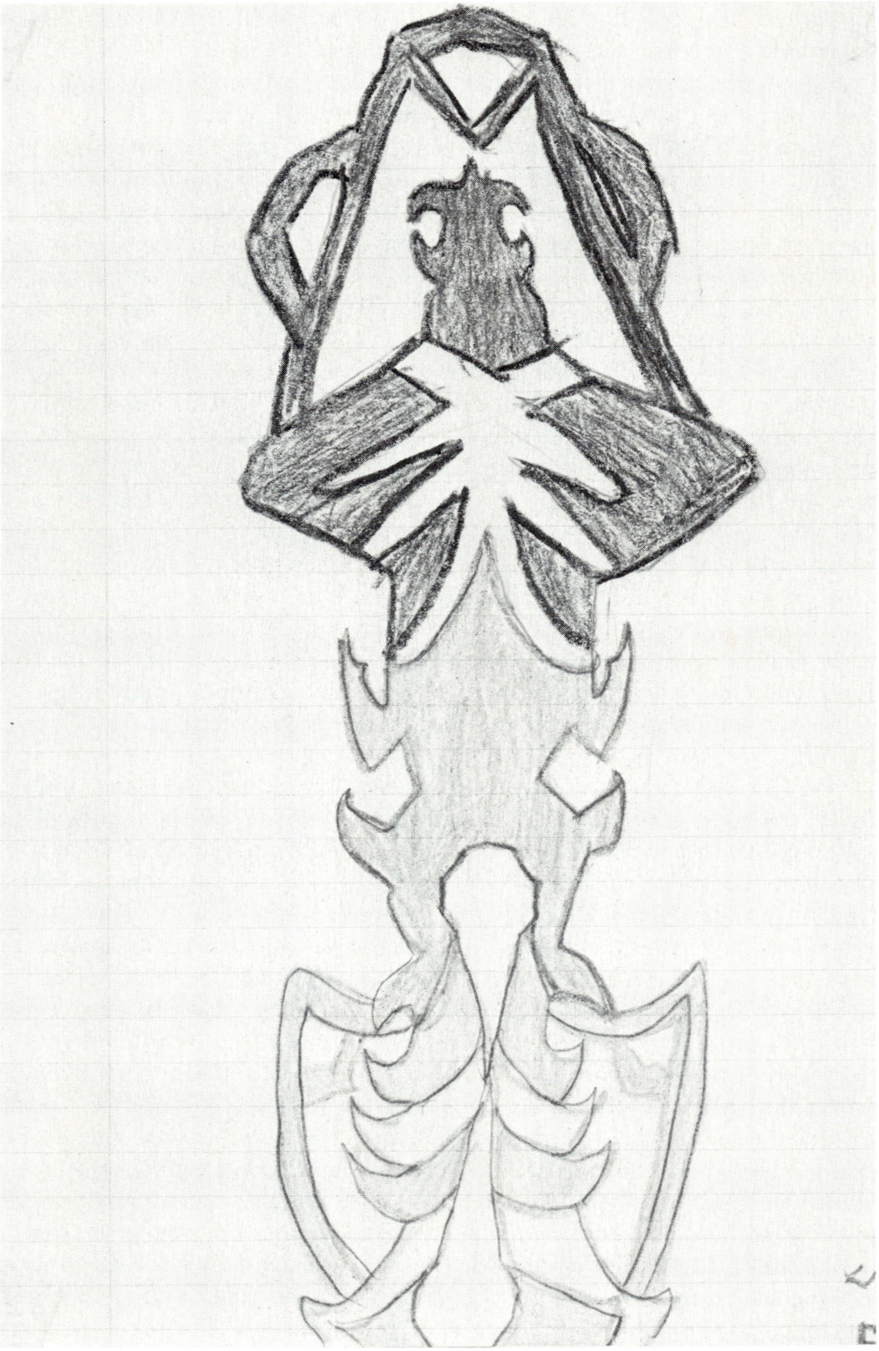

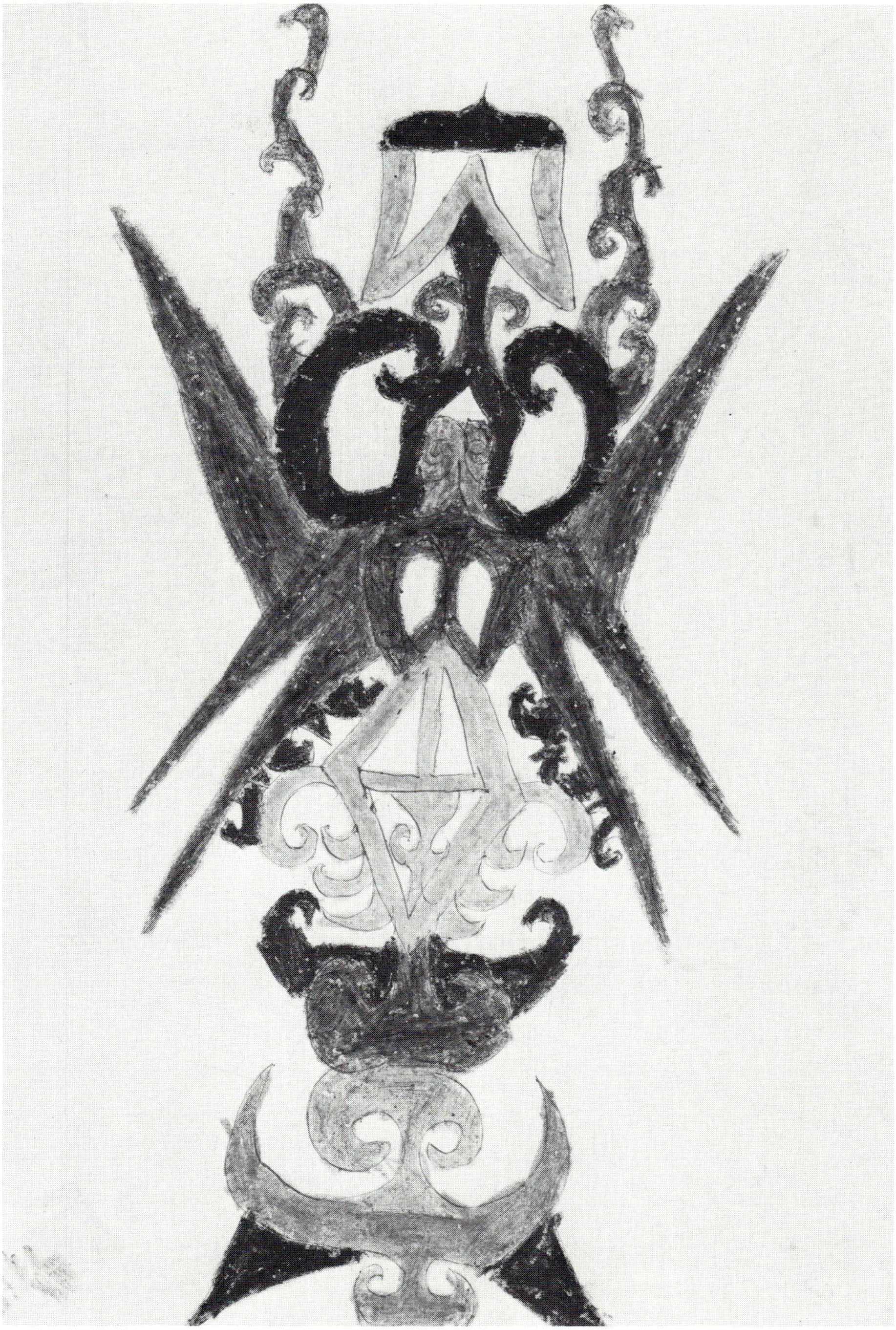

II

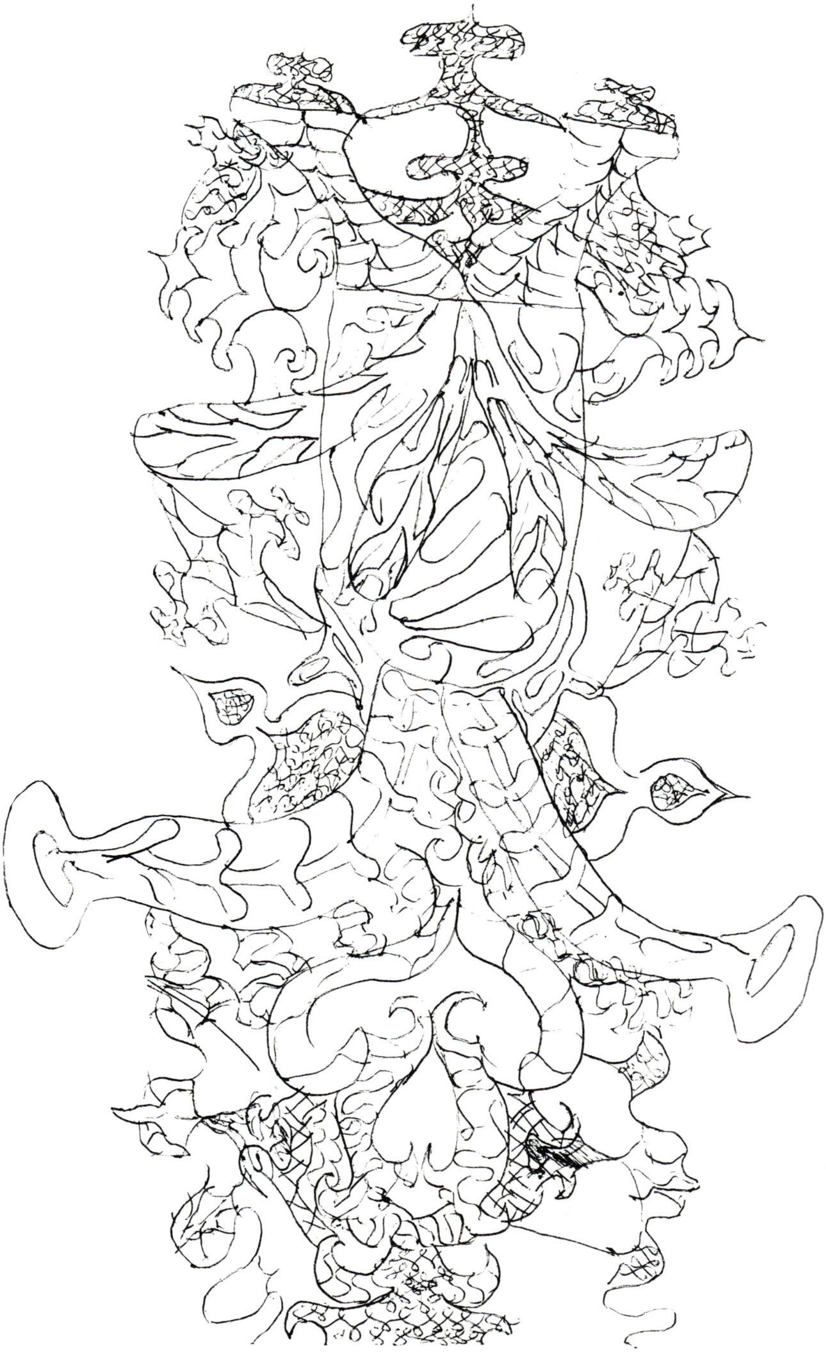

III

The stench surrounding Doreen deepened. She had given up washing, and paradoxically, she seemed much happier. She started to munch cookies in the therapist's presence but warded off all attempts at discovering what it might mean to eat in one's therapist's presence. Like a little savage, she would hurriedly stuff her mouth, turned away from the therapist, and then set about her routine of hopping, skipping and jumping. She indicated with gestures and facial expressions that the therapist was to approve of this wholeheartedly. About the only thing that could interrupt her unflagging pursuit of pleasure and tension release was a verbal interpretation that included mention of a body part. This would activate the tic and make Doreen repeat her warnings not to look at it.

On occasion, she would stop herself in her physical activities and tell yet another vignette of the continuous marital battles of her parents which they had almost daily. She told of running between them, trying to shield mother from father's blows, and father from mother's screaming. She told of locking herself into the bathroom and hiding under her bed, until the need to run away became so deep it was transformed into her mode of being-in-the-world and daydreaming withdrawal took the place of living. Eventually, she also told of her deep dismay at being unable to control either her surroundings or her body. All this while, her motility and her behavior at home remained regressive and infantile.

In the sessions, she revealed herself as a child who had somatized the anxiety caused by repeated trauma in an attempt to recapture and never give up the fleeting satisfaction of being mother's baby; hence the inability to acknowledge the beauty of her young girl's body and the lack of bladder control. Instead of emotions and feelings, she appeared to experience various musculatory, respiratory and circulating sensations, which, when strong, culminated in the aforementioned tic. The treatment approach was to allow Doreen to rebuild her self-image under the benevolent influence of a strong positive transference for the therapist so that her ego might gain sufficient reintegration of motor function and body sensation to allow for assimilation of word concepts describing these actions and feelings.

After a prolonged period of acting out her need to be someone's loved baby, and keeping the environment at bay by her unattractive appearance and behavior, Doreen began to "act in—" solely within the therapeutic hour. That is, consistent approving reflections in her therapist's eyes, physical mirroring of her movement and consistent verbal transference interpretations brought about this change. Doreen gave up her provacative and manipulative withdrawal at home and in school at about the same time she began to use the therapist's bathroom frequently. This was discussed in terms of her wanting to please, rather than being pleased by others. She, in her turn, started to talk about the function of liquid—as a drink, a fertilizer, a discharge, etc. The wetness and smell of her sheets after she had urinated into them, as well as their displeasing coldness which often awoke her, also came into focus. Eventually, she gained permission from her mother to change her sheets herself, provided she washed them out after use.

The recognition of her own body functions appeared to permit her to recognize other, more abstract functions, as well. The day came when she asked if wetting her bed were also a "running away." In answer to a request for clarification she said she wet her bed instead of hitting her mother.

Her interests suddenly turned to the arts. She began to ask questions about various forms of dance in identification with her therapist and began to draw pictures of dances. (See pictures p. 108) Her improvisations became structured replays of felt experiences, exhibiting both exu-

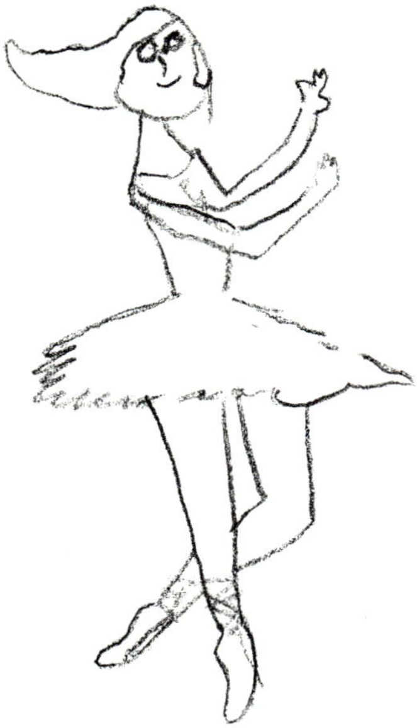

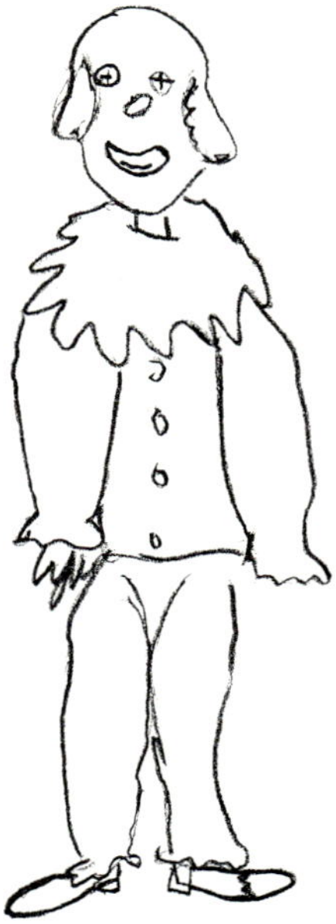

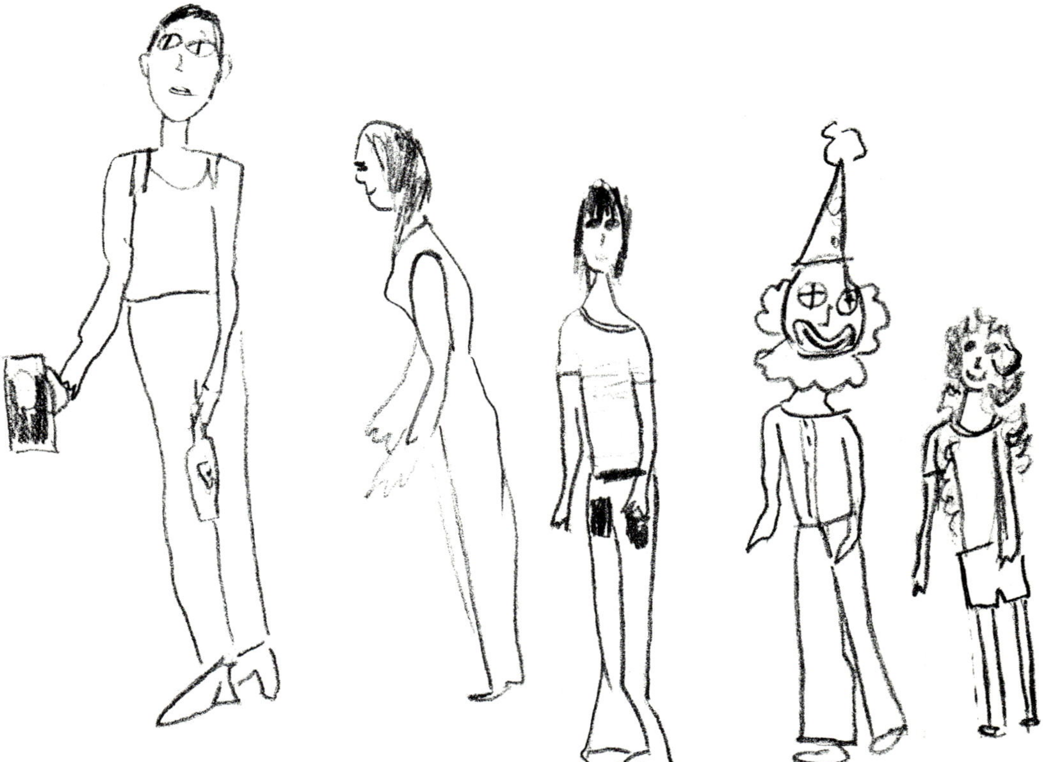

berance and control of space. The tortured rigidities and tensions disappeared like an unwanted scaffolding although the tic and the headaches had not been specifically analyzed either verbally or nonverbally. With the growth of a healthy body image and the conscious acceptance of inner body sensitivities as meaningful signals, Doreen no longer had to act the smelly, uncontrolled monster. In moods of self-derision rather than depression, she decided to portray herself as a clown. A family drawing accurately portrayed the mother turned away from the children to the husband who holds a bottle and a beer glass. Doreen had become capable of facing her own reality, indeed, without flinching from it.

Significantly, she did not tell her mother that the enuresis had been cleared up. Her mother, however, noticed that the need for sheets had dwindled. She promptly withdrew Doreen from treatment, without permitting a resolution of the transference situation, or indeed, without regard for Doreen's still vulnerable sense of self.

In summary: Doreen's treatment, which had indeed only lasted the predicted one year, followed the usual process of initial improvement, regression to the fixation point and conflict resolution expected in this form of treatment.

Primary treatment tools were a combination of verbal transference interpretations and dance movement structured to conform to the developmental levels of the patient. Symptom alleviation, as well as some conflict resolution occurred when object related motility became a felt and integrated reality.

Bibliography

American Psychoanalytic Association. *A Glossary of Psychoanalytic Terms and Concepts.* New York: APA, 1971.

Bernstein, P. *Theory and Methods in Dance-movement Therapy.* Dubuque: Kendall/Hunt, 1972.

Fenichel, O. *The Psychoanalytic Theory of Neurosis.* New York: Norton & Co., 1945.

Friedman, L. "The Therapeutic Alliance," International Journal of Psychoanalysis, #50, 139, 1969.

Glover, E. *On the Early Development of the Mind.* London: Imago Publishing Co., 1956.

Greenacre, Phyllis. "The Predisposition to Anxiety," *The Psychoanalytic Quarterly,* Vol. X, No. 1.

Hartman H. *Ego Psychology and the Problem of Adaptation.* New York: International University Press, 1958.

Hoffer, W. "Mouth, Hand and Ego Integration," *Psychoanalytic Study of the Child,* Vol. 3/4, New York: International University Press, 1949.

———. "Development of the Body Ego," *Psychoanalytic Study of the Child,* Vol 5., New York: International University Press, 1950.

Heidegger, M. *Being and Time.* New York: Harper & Rowe, 1962.

Jacobson, Edith. *The Self and the Object World.* New York: International University Press, 1964.

Kestenberg, Judith. "The Role of Movement Patterns in Development," *Psychoanalytic Quarterly,* New York, 1967.

Lowen, A. *The Betrayal of the Body.* London: Collier MacMillan, Ltd., 1967.

Mahler, Margaret *On Human Symbiosis and the Vicissitudes of Individuation.* New York: International University Press, 1968.

Reich, W. *Character Analysis.* New York: Farrar Strauss and Cudahy, 1949.

Schilder, P. *The Image and Appearance of the Human Body.* New York: International University Press, 1950.

———. *Contributions to Developmental Neuropsychiatry.* New York: International University Press, 1964.

Schur, M. "Comments on the Metapsychology of Somatization," *Psychoanalytic Study of the Child.* New York: International University Press, 1955.

Siegel, Elaine and Blau, Bette. "Breathing Together"—a preliminary investigation of a motor reflex as adaptation—variability of Forced Vital Capacity in Psychotic Children. Unpublished research paper.
Siegel, Elaine V. "Psyche and Soma: Movement Therapy," *Voices,* Special Issue, Skokie, Ill., 1970.
———. "Movement Therapy with Autistic Children," *Psychoanalytic Review,* Vol. 60, #1, 1973.
———. "Movement Therapy as a Psychoanalytic Tool," Journal of the American Psychoanalytic Association. Vol. 21, #2, 1973.
———. "Psychoanalytic Thought and Methodology in Dance/Movement Therapy," *Focus on Dance.* VII, AAHPER, Washington, D.C.
———. *Desomatization and How to Effect It.* Tape series, Behavioral Sciences Tape Library, Leonia, N.J.
Silverman, I. "Two types of Preoedipal Character Disorders," *International Journal of Psychoanalysis,* #38, 1957.
Spitz, R. *The First Year of Life.* New York: International University Press, 1965.

Chapter 8

THE USE OF SYMBOLISM WITHIN A GESTALT MOVEMENT THERAPY APPROACH

*Penny Lewis Bernstein, Ph.D., DTR**

Genesis

Since I feel strongly that my evolution as a dance-movement therapist has as much to do with my own personal growth, as it has with my training and work with clients; I will be sharing my concerns from the viewpoints of a spiritual pilgrim, client, and therapist. From these perspectives, I have grown to respect the power of allowing unintegrated parts of an individual's being to live fully in an accepting non-judgemental manner. Early on in my college life I had been involved in verbal therapy. Using intellectualization as my primary defense I was readily able to discuss at length my fears and angers, analyze from whence they came, and thereby assume I could dispense with both affect and conflict. Of course, that did not occur; and unfortunately, the verbal psychotherapist did not have the tools at his disposal to facilitate my tapping into and exploring those hidden pockets of emotional crisis. Only when I came in contact with the body therapies did I begin an integration process and take the first steps toward becoming a human "being."

The concept that became so clear to me that I have since incorporated into my work with others is, that growth is more apt to take place if an individual is involved in the experience they are feeling rather than just talking about it. It is important to live the experience, "participate" in it as the Polster's describe it—as if it were happening in the here and now (Polster & Polster, 1973). And, in fact, if the person allows this enactment to involve his total being; the "as if" dissipates, and there is a full identification with the process.

I have found also that when the drama is allowed to occur without having the parent-top dog rear its demanding judgemental head, integration can occur more readily. Caustic comments such as, "Oh this is silly, you're acting foolish" or "You better stop doing this or someone will put you away" or "Don't you show this part of you; its hideous; people won't like you; they'll reject you for sure," keep a person from experiencing himself as a totality.

A supportive caring environment is needed in order to facilitate a self trust. External as well as internal acceptance is paramount. If I, as therapist, can let that person know that I have utmost respect for *all* of his being—including and most particularly those hidden, darkened places; he may be able to begin to risk knowing a little more of himself. If I can help him to be aware of his critic and the role it plays in inhibiting the union or reunion of his being, he may begin to accept even the non-accepting aspect of himself and let it be through an infinitely tolerant observing self.

This very same non-judgemental observer self is a concept which is active in my spiritual evolution as well. During meditation, whether I am sitting or moving such as with conscious

*Penny Bernstein holds a diploma in gestalt therapy. She is the Administrative Coordinator for the Antioch-New England Graduate school masters in movement therapy program and is engaged in private practice.

walking or T'ai Chi, I am trying to clear my thoughts of "mind dust" without punishing myself for my inability to maintain quietude. Alan Watts wrote on meditation:

> As you pursue that experiment you will very naturally find that you can' help naming sounds, identifying them, and go on thinking, talking to yourself inside your head, automatically. But it's important that you don't try to repress those thoughts by forcing them out of your mind because that will have precisely the same effect as if you were trying to smooth rough water with a flat iron—you're just going to disturb it all the more. What you do is this: as you hear sounds coming into your head, or thoughts, you simply listen to them as part of general noise going on just as you would be listening to cars going by, or to birds chattering outside the window. So look at your own thoughts as just noises. And soon you will find that the outside world and the inside world come together. They are a happening just like the sounds going on outside, and all you are doing is watching it (1974, p. 29).

Watts speaks of the union of the outside and inside world. My feeling is that before a "transcendental union" can occur that an "internal union" must take place. The few times in my life that I have experienced Satori, i.e., that I have allowed myself an awareness of my unity with the cosmos, I have gone through a process whereby my judgemental self is at peace. How I am, my essence, separate from any roles that my parent tells me I have to play, emerges. I am at one with myself. I am me, nondefined, and thus not limited to any behavior. My accepting observer is free to SEE fully while my body is equally free to experience the omnipotent orgasm which transpires when I am at one with the All.

As I share this experience I am reminded how my spiritual beliefs concur and harmonize with my professional philosophic approach. Coming from a generation which has so acutely observed the split between the spiritual and mundane lives of many, I cannot work any other way. Simply, I want for myself to allow myself the serenity that is within the nature of surrendering to and accepting that which exists. I feel one of the most important tenets in both the process toward spiritual unity and personal unity, is the concept of staying in the present.

A person may be said to be a a spiritual standstill if he plagues himself with the past or the future. The only time that exists is the *present,* and the only way to reach Satori is through immersion in the now. Time has no existence in and of itself, it is only a concept which has been created by man. Being totally aware of what exists in the present, both internally and externally, is the doorway to experiencing what exists in other levels of reality including the most basic: the eternal now—pure energy.

One of the primary tenets of Gestalt therapy is the maintaining of an awareness of the here and now. "What are you feeling now?" is a question often asked by the therapist. Power resides in experiencing the present rather than talking about something that has happened or may happen. Both past and future as well as present can be experienced in the now in a therapeutic experiment; thus there is no need for separation of feeling or action. This awareness extends also to the outside environment. Seeing, hearing, tasting, touching, and even smelling are all sensing processes which gestaltists encourage individuals to explore more fully. Perls, Hefferline and Goodman, in *Gestalt Therapy* (1965) suggest countless experiments designed to heighten sensory awareness. To sense more fully the natural environment has led me into spiritual unions as joyful as anything that I have ever experienced.

As I speak of union, I know also that oneness or integration is an ongoing never-ending process; and part of the process for me both as client and therapist has been the acknowledgement of the disunity and disharmony that exists within most human beings. As with a child's game, the only place to begin is at "GO"; the rules are that you can't start in the middle. When a person becomes aware of the many separate and usually conflictual aspects of himself and begins to emphasize and crystallize the opposing thoughts and wants, he has started on the journey toward internal harmony. Stressing his disunity may seem to draw him further away from this goal to some; but in actuality, I have found that it is only in encouraging these conflictual parts to be fully manifested and expressed, that they will every be evolved into quietude within the self. This process seems to occur only when the whole body is involved in the experiment. This means that the head, which often harbors the judging self and the intellect (a highly valued aspect of an individual's being—so deeply enthroned that it often rules to the exclusion of the sensuous feeling self) does not try to subvert the enactment, but rather is involved in it. Blocks elsewhere in the body must subside whether they be in the form of tense body armor (Reich, 1949), numbed limpness, or dissynchronous movement. Breathing also must be allowed to be in service to the movement ritual that is taking place.

Basic to Gestalt therapy theory is the concept of figure-ground relationship—bringing into awareness and experience "shadowy pockets" of unresolved conflicts. Clarifying the diverse parts often facilitates a decision making process. E.g., "Should I stay in college or free myself of academia?" Parent: "You do what you are supposed to and you are supposed to go to college" versus child: "I want to play and feel free and have fun." It can also allow someone to be in touch with and carry out a basic need; e.g., "I want to be loved and cared for, therefore I an going to risk being open and vulnerable."

I have shared how I have grown to value the importance of experiencing with the total being, unintegrated parts of the self, of observing and non-judgementally accepting this process through a supportive environment, of maintaining awareness in the now, and, finally, of emphasizing and personifying the conflicted and often polarized feelings so as to clarify the figure from the background, thus facilitating resolution and integration.

Now I would like to share the utmost respect I have for the symbolic process within each individual. Early in my professional career as an occupational therapist, I facilitated a task-oriented group of hospitalized psychiatric patients. The task they had decided upon was the construction of a doll house for the pediatric ward. During its construction, one of the men continually expressed a fear that the house was going to collapse. I responded through reality testing by pointing out how the nails were adequately placed and the materials strong. This never seemed to alter his perception and fear, however. It was only when I realized that the house symbolized both the evolving group and his feeling regarding his inner state that I was able to really hear and respond to him. When I spoke with him utilizing his symbols, we were truly communicating with each other and experiencing contact. Growth seemed to occur more rapidly, until, as trust developed, I was able to mirror his concerns in secondary process language. So by the time the project was completed he exclaimed, "You know, I think this doll house is pretty sturdy." "Yes," I said, "Our group seems to be durable too. We've been with each other through a lot. We've been helpful to each other and to ourselves and can feel our strengths more and more." "Yeh," he said, with a knowing smile.

In my study and work in dance therapy, I have tapped into and made use of my own as well as others unconscious symbolism. It is often scary to zero in on causes of conflict or targets of anger. It is far easier to make use of an individual's symbolic processes. Although children's symbols are more readily available through their fantasy dramas, adults too have access to primary process material. Dreams have consistently been avenues into the darkened caverns of the unconscious; however, ritualized habitual patterns of movement have been the doorway for many into more deeper awareness of themselves. Jung, the father of the therapeutic exploration of symbolism, made use of this medium. He cites occasions when he had clients "dance their unconscious figures" (1968). This process of allowing an individual's total being to become immersed in the expression of the unconscious—not just talking about, but fully experiencing the symbols—affords him direct contact with parts of his being which he may have previously disowned or of which he has been unaware. Observing the "demon," as one client named him, emerge from a seemingly quiet hollowed, narrowed body was for me a beautiful ritual. His eyes, once meek and subdued, glowed with fiery energy. His breathing increased and spread, for the first time in therapy, throughout his whole body. Hissing and growling at the group, he moved merging gesture with posture, crawling, leaping with agility, and clawing at members who didn't respond with respect. He had previously never fully given vent to the more aggressive evil side of his being. Having denied its existence, he had never fully accepted this part of himself. When goodness exists, evil, as its polarity, is also present. I feel it important to accept my own potential for doing harm. If I do not, in a symbolic way, I have given my power to this unresolved part. Once I respect that, like its antithesis, the capacity for evil is within me; my total self is then in control of this "demon." Thus, I own my evil instead of it owning me.

Feelings such as anger, sadness, and fear can also be symbolically personified. And if they have been previously repressed, they too may have been fantasized as having overwhelming omnipotence by the individual; e.g., "My God, if I ever really get angry, I'll kill everyone in this room." or "If I ever allow myself to really cry, I'll stay in a funk for the rest of my life and never do anything again."

With a constructive environment, the person can give vent to this aspect of himself and allow this symbolic expression to become not just unconsciously, but consciously real.

Once the latter process transpires the person becomes closer to targeting his emotion, e.g., "At whom am I angry?" or "What is my loss?" And once targeted, he is well on his way to accepting his right to feel and thus integrating his unresolved gestalt.

Finally, for me, one of the most important understandings which I have grown to appreciate not only as a therapist but as one involved in both personal and transpersonal growth, is the value of and sensitivity to one's internal rhythm. Barry Stevens, a well known Gestaltist, wrote a book aptly titled *Don't Push the River.* I have learned, sometimes painfully, that *I can't push the river.*

Each individual has his own inner timing for growth. I, myself, vacillate between diving into working with a conflict and wading slowly, getting immersed in the therapeutic process a step at a time. But I have grown to know that I can't "dive in" if my rhythm says to "go slow with this one." I have found also that even when an individual takes a surprising step and plunges over his head; he "forgets" what transpired in the session until he is ready to integrate it. One such individual claimed that she was "not herself." (We are who we are.) What happened was that not being familiar with the power of movement she was not as heavily defensed as she was verbally; and although she claimed the experience was a positive one for her at the time, she had difficulty integrating this new found sensation and perception of herself. In her subsequent sessions I structured the experiments in such a way as to provide a synchrony between her internal rhythm and her process of growth. And as she trusted more and more, she began to risk taking larger steps into the murky waters of the unknown.

Theoretical Model

Concepts

Gestalt Movement Therapy

Any holistic present-oriented use of body awareness and movement directed toward the grounded integration of dissociated areas of an individual through the facilitation of spontaneous figure formation and organismic self-regulation toward expressive contact with the environment.

Movement Experiment

An improvisation involving the body designed to explore the unintegrated part(s) of an individual. In most instances this involves the approach of previously avoided material.

Gestalt

A form that cannot be broken down without its own destruction; take a successfully completed movement out of a dance composition and it ceases to exist as a work of art.

Movement Therapy

Any therapeutic use of movement directed toward the physical and psychic integration of the individual. (ADTA) The body and the mind are not separate aspects of a person's being. When they are experienced as such, "My head is where it's at. My intelligence and calm logic is what should be in control. And my body with all its base animalistic feelings exists only to serve my objective commands," a person is not experiencing a sense of oneness with himself. The use of movement, along with its cognitive counterpart, can provide a vehicle for the reintegration or reunion of an individual's being.

Holism

The principle that an organism is not equal to the sum of its parts and must be studied as a whole. An individual is composed of many discernable parts: a brain, a stomach, muscles, etc. If explored and treated separately, a verbally oriented psychiatrist would study his brain; a physical therapist his tense muscles; an internist his stomach ulcer; they will all render the individual a gross injustice. Even if they consulted with each other, the man is more than just all these parts put together. There is a special gestalt—that of the man with all of his being interacting within and without. This organismic integrity provides an interactive system. What effects a part of a person sets in motion a whole chain of responses.* Likewise, a group is more than just the sum of its members. There are group issues which would not exist without its membership. In addition, group accommodations, compensations, rigidities can evolve from the influence of one member, i.e., one can cause repercussion on the total functioning.

Present-oriented Therapy

An approach which stresses the maintenance of a here and now awareness emphasizing the experience of behavior as it is sensed. The technique of a continuum of awareness exemplifies use of this concept in Gestalt Therapy: The client is asked repeatedly to finish the sentence, "Now I am feeling . . ."

*Because of this natural interconnection, it is vital to "replace" any aspect of the individual with which one works into the total entity to sense the relationships and effects on the rest of his functionings.

Figure-background Formation

Background is the undifferentiated field, the emerging focus is the figure (Latner, 1973). The ability to clarify the figure from the background provides a figure background formation. For example, a person may be looking for another individual in a crowd. He scans the grouping of people, finding the individual he then fixes his gaze on her. The rest of the crowd becomes field or background, while she, the object of his focus, becomes the figure. He sees her clearly while the others are blurred from his heightened awareness of her presence. Likewise, an individual may feel physically uncomfortable but not have focused on what is causing this discomfort. He may become aware of the fact that although he is supposedly resting in a relaxed manner, his neck muscles are quite tense. His head is being held and is not fully giving in to its weight. In the instant of this awareness, the figure of his tense neck muscles and held head comes into focus while the rest of his environment both internal and exernal drifts from consciousness and forms a background. A gestalt formation has occured. He now has an opportunity to further explor this figure, thereby providing a means to integrate those feelings which have produced or been stored in his bound body.

Organismic Self-regulation

This concept entails the innate capacity for a living creature to strive toward homeostatic equilibrium. Common to all animate beings is the life process of constantly requiring substances from its environment in order to exist. Being able to be aware of needs: nourishment, elimination, sexual gratification, shelter, etc., and to take on the responsibility of having those needs met, is part of being a functioning adult. As a neonate, much of the responsibility of having those needs satisfied is or should exist within the environment. The parent or surrogate parent feeds and cares for the infant. As the child matures, he assumes more and more of the responsibility for meeting his own needs and for actively seeking a suitable environment which will provide the required elements for his homostasis and self-actualization.

In order for this process to occur fully, all of the individual's ego must be syntonic or in agreement with the need satisfying behavior. If, for example, he seeks sexual gratification with a woman, and part of him tells him that "women will envelop you and castrate you"; he is not coming from an integrated unified stance. He will not be able to fully satisfy his need; part of him will be fearful and angry. He will not be able to experience ejaculation, phallic sadistic rather than genital rhythms may be used during coitus, as well as numerous body blocks of the experience of orgasm.*

Spontaneous Figure Formation

Another aspect of functioning behavior, spontaneous figure formation, involves the capacity to allow the process of needs and feelings to be brought into conscious focus as they come into existence. This requires the ability to be fully and acceptingly aware of and responsible for personal

**Phallic-aggressive rhythms*. This involves the ability to control phallic-aggressive rhythms which characterize leaps and the ballistic qualities in most sports activities. (Kestenberg, 1967, Bernstein, 1975) On a flow line it is characterized by high intensity, sharp flow adjustment with steep increases and decreases in tension.

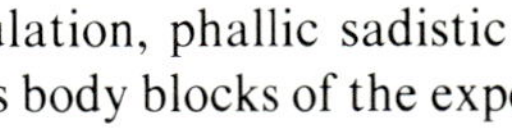

Phallic-inner genital rhythms. This involves the ability to combine and control phallic and inner genital rhythms. (Marcus and Kestenberg) It is the predominating characteristic genital rhythm of normal adults and graphed on a flow line, it is characterized by medium intensity rounded transitions. (Kestenbery, 1967, Bernstein, 1975)

behavior. This is a "process of creative adjustments that come through the formulation and destruction of gestalts" (Latner, 1973).

The other aspect of this process is the ability to allow the gestalts once formed and responded to, to be destroyed, i.e., drift back into subliminal awareness within the background. "Figure-ground reversibility (what is being discussed here) is at the root of fluidity in life" claim the Polsters (Polster & Polster, 1973).

Contact

The ability to fully experience a contingency or confrontation between two separate entities is another aspect of functional behavior. The Polsters define contact as "a dynamic relationship occuring only at the boundaries of two compellingly attractive but clearly differentiated figures of interest" (Polster & Polster, 1973, p. 107). This can exist between the self and another or among parts of the individual. For example, a person may become aware of how tense his shoulders and upper arms are, rendering his upper extremities ineffectual in any action requiring the use of dynamic movement. As the figures emerge from the field, he realizes that one muscle system may want to strike out and feel anger while the other opposing contracting system may want to control this expression. Feeling anger may be seen as being bad and unlovable. When these two figures confront each other fully and clearly, they are experiencing contactfulness.

Groundedness

Another quality which is part of a functioning human is that of groundedness. This concept may be defined as the process of being centered (Latner, 1973). This essentially involves the proper alignment of the body with a capacity to allow energy to flow throughout the total body. Groundedness also implies a capacity to function within reality,* to take responsibility for existence, at any given moment in time. A balanced, grounded, centered body means a balanced centered psyche.

Theoretical Formulations

Method of Identification

"In sickness men have types, in health all are unique" (Perls, Hefferline, Goodman, 1965). Because Gestalt therapy has traditionally moved away from the medical model, diagnosis** as is usually conceptualized is non-existent. No categories are affixed to the individual, rather it is the patterns of behavior which are explored. Latner writes:

> "Diagnosis in Gestalt Therapy is underlining the patterns of the patient's behavior and of his interactions with the therapist. In the course of therapy as the patient changes, the characteristics change. He is not stuck forever with a label, for the label does not refer to some unchanging parts of his psyche as traditional psychodiagnostic labels do, but to current behavior and attitudes." (1973)

Fagan (1970) refers to this concept as the "process of patterning." When a client states his goals or a symptom of which he wishes to be freed, the therapist begins to assist that person in

*The ground or earth is often considered symbolic of reality, e.g., "he had his feet on the ground."

**Diagnosis—Classification of individuals on the basis of observed symptoms or characteristics and usually abnormalities (Wolman, 1975).

becoming aware of the here-now behavior which holds him in the habitual non-spontaneous non-need-satisfying way of responding.

For example, a young college woman was referred to me for help. Her goals, now realized were: "I want to find out who I am so that I can feel comfortable about myself and therefore feel comfortable around other people. I want to feel secure and independent. I want to be happier. I hate being depressed all the time. I want to like myself and other people."

When I first saw her, she had no recollection of the first twelve years of her life. Her memories of her childhood began after the death of her mother who had been ill consistently throughout her early years. At the time of her therapy Beth was living in a commune feeling rejected by all but her loving, highly defensed boyfriend. As we progressed in therapy it became clear that she had a deep feeling of separateness and anger toward Diane, the unnamed head of the household. Concommitant with these feelings was a relentless desire to be "close" with her. She began to see her habitual spatial and body posturing behavior toward Diane, as well as others in her surrogate family, in relation to her unmet needs and blocked expressions during her childhood. Part of her growth and subsequent termination came when Beth was able to relate to Diane and others on a here-now basis, seeing Diane as Diane and clarifying her own needs and from whence they came.

As with Beth, most dysfunctional behavior occurs when there are unresolved gestalts often caused by childhood unfinished business. Unintegrated figure formations such as these are never fully suppressed, however; and the individual continues to behave as if the conflict is still happening. Her daily existence is spent in attempts to relive and satisfy unfulfilled needs. This is a never-ending endeavor as no environment can ever be exactly like the one in the past. And no new figure formation can emerge if the background contains these unresolved gestalts. Thus real awareness of the present is negated, and her behavior becomes habitual, mechanistic, and rigid.

There are several approaches that I have found to be most effective in assisting an individual and therby myself in becoming more aware of himself and his habitual body patterning. The following are a few examples:

Sense awareness body journey: One of the most widely utilized experiments is the awareness journey. In this instance the therapist directs a sense exploration for the individual. I suggest that the person or persons find a comfortable place on the floor and lie on their backs. I usually play a recording of some white noise; I like the ocean as it replicates the breath process. I suggest also that they turn their awareness inward looking inside their body and hearing their internal sounds.

"Can you feel each toe and its position without having to move it? . . . Sense your temperature, the texture and pressure of clothing around you or where the air is in contact with your skin and where your toes touch each other;" etc., etc., until the whole body is covered.

Breathing is also centered upon. Individuals are asked to outline the breath flow within their torso. Connections are then made to those areas which are felt less than others, numb spots, areas that tingle, are cold, or in pain. These places, too, are mapped out exactly in the body.

Although I am quite often aware of these areas upon initial observation; it is vital that the individual himself identify them. Therefore, I take my cues from him; *he* tells me and our work toward a more free and adaptively spontaneous body begins.

The body talks: Another approach which I am finding to be quite effective is a different form of a body journey. The former was in a way a more passive approach. In this instance, the therapist is a silent listener. The client is asked to find a position which is both familiar and comfortable to him. He is then asked to exaggerate the pattern, e.g., becoming more tensely bound or flaccid, moving to a more close or open position. He is then asked to take a trip inside his body and to speak from each part that wants to say something.

Beth, the young women, mentioned earlier responded:

"I am Beth's legs. I want to run away.

I am Beth's hands. I am making a fist and want to punch out.

I am Beth's head, I make sure I keep her confused.

I am her voice. I am weak like a child's.

I am her heart . . . broken."

And then finally, "I am Beth's tears, I am sad. . . ."

Immediately prior to this experiment, Beth had been running around in confused circles rambling from her head without any awareness or contact with her body and her hidden feelings.

Gestalt and Massage: On occasion an individual needs assistance in becoming aware of his body patterning. Massage, with its "laying on of hands" also serves to generate a more positive energy flow with the passage of energy from the therapist to the client. Massage also says to that person that as his therapist I am capaple of caring for and accepting him through the most primary avenue of communication: the human touch.*

Here again the individual is asked to speak from the part of the body centered upon. However, in this instance, the therapist with her observing eye can select the initial area of concern. Places for attention may be: areas in the torso where breathing is curtailed, parts which feel tense or cold to the touch, joints which are not aligned, areas which have an unproportional amount of muscle or fat, or others which seem lifeless and limp.

Jane, a client, whose work was brief and profound began talking from her lower back which had seemed held and unaligned with the rest of her spine.

"I am Jane's back, I'm tight. I'm not going to let her feel any of those things she's not supposed to . . ."

From there, I took my cues from her. She became aware of her thighs tensing and tingling. We moved the massage and attention to them.

"I am Jane's thighs," she reported. "I work with the lower back to keep Jane from feeling . . ."

Her leg abductors, too, were tense. They spoke as did her breathing as being "locked out" of her pelvis.

Therapy began with the initially quiet but adamant emergence of the sensual Jane, teaming up with her breathing process. Once the figures emerged with their corresponding body patterns; she could begin to work through and resolve her sexual conflict and accept more fully her right to womanhood and aggression.

Identification through patterns of movement: There are several methods which I utilize which assist in the identification of habitual movement patterns. Here are a few:

Body walking postures: I have the individual walk in his usual manner. After having observed the body posture for a period of time, I exaggerate the imbalanced non-adaptive patterns by placing the individual or suggesting to him to move his body a certain way. Muscles can become more bound or limp, his body shape more open or shrunken.

*The use of touch is both a powerful and potentially destructive tool. Issues such as sexuality and countertransference must not be overlooked.

He then is asked to resume walking once more, this time paying close attention to what he is feeling moment to moment. "Gee, I really lead with my chin." or "I feel afraid to touch the ground" have been comments which have assisted individuals in a growth process.

Effort-shape exaggeration: As I have studied, effort-shape, a system of movement observation and notation devised by Rudolf Laban and Warren Lamb, I make use of the simple conceptual breakdown of the dynamics of movement and the shape the patterns take in space (Bernstein, 1975). With this system in hand it is fairly easy to grasp an individual's body attitude or favorite effort combination during an experiment which explores various environments and movement combinations. Once again, it is the individual himself who identifies those dance-like patterns which are more comfortable, more familiar to him. When these dynamic combinations are exaggerated figure formation can readily occur.

One woman darted around the studio, winding indirectly and circling the therapist. Her head in the air, she gently propelled her body upwards and away from the floor. From this experience she came in contact with her intense fear of committment and of the "violation" of involvement with others. She became aware of her familiar pattern of "circling" groups and issues, never being able to be a part and stop long enough to risk taking a stand.

Awareness of recurrent patterns: Even without the use of effor-shape, recurring gestures and postural patterns can easily be centered upon.

For example: "I am Jim's foot. I am tense and cocked ready to push you away. You're coming too close and I won't permit you to get close to Jim or Jim to be close with you." Or:

"I am rocking the little girl in Celest, I take care of her when she feels sad and keep her from feeling too bad. I have to keep her quiet." And finally, to Celeste's child: "You shut up you little obnoxious baby! You're always crying for something, you're never satisfied!"

Therapeutic Process

With a goal of awakening awareness and a maintaining of a present oriented, free contactful grounded body, not cramped by the past or crippled by future expectations; the Gestalt therapeutic process revolves around the ability to formulate figures spontaneously. Simply this process may be outlined as follows:

1. Awareness of and identification on non-adaptive patterns of behavior, e.g., habitual body tension, restricted natural breath process, or dominance of a particular movement sequence or dynamic.
2. Crystallization of conflictual parts, e.g., "I have tension on the back of my neck; my head wants to rule without having my body sensations interrupt its logical functioning; my body with all my locked feelings demands to be released and integrated."
3. Experiencing choice, e.g., "If I want I can really indulge the child in me and giggle and cry without having to analyze it."
4. Figure formation—the reaching of clarity and experiencing the gestalt, e.g., "We can work together. There can be a time for you and me." Feelings to head: "I like your strength and intelligence." Head to body: "I like your warmth and fun and ability to be close with other people."
5. Destruction of a figure. Upon owning that part, the individual relaxes as the figure moves into subliminal awareness.

6. Creative indifference. The individual is then in an open here-now awareness state ready for a new gestalt formation.

There are numerous gestalt techniques, some have already been menioned in their relationship to initial figure identification process. Here are just a few:

1. Awareness continuum: As the person is stationery or moving, suggest to him to continuously complete the following phrase, "Now I am aware of . . ."
2. Repeating: Suggest to the individual to repeat a gesture or movement pattern which seems to be authentic or habitual for them.
3. Exaggeration: Suggest to the individual to exaggerate a gesture, movement, or breathing process. This may take the form of intensifying the movement dynamics used such as strength or lightness, quickness or slowness, directness or indirectness; enlarging upon the shape of the pattern; or evolving the sequence from a solely gestural to a postural movement encompassing the whole body.*
4. Verbalization in service of the body: Making a sound from a tense area or movement sequence can often aid in the gestalt formulation. An individual may not be able to identify the blocked body feeling, however once a sound, be it noise or gibberish, is made and repeated during exhalation; emotion readily surfaces.

   Or, suggestions such as "Give words to your movement." "If your gesture could talk, what would it say?" "Give a voice to your feeling, be that feeling." Or "What would your (body part) say to you (other body part or somaticized defense)?"
5. Feeding of a pattern: The therapist may "feed" the individual a movement pattern or verbal phrase for the individual to explore. For example, the therapist might suggest to an individual with tense buttocks and locked knees and legs to stamp his feet asserting "no" in a reciprocal "yes-no" dyad with the therapist.
6. Reversals: The therapist may suggest to the individual to reverse the movement pattern or postural figuration. The concept of polarization is used often in Gestalt therapy. The feeling is that if one part of an individual's personality functions strongly; its opposite is present as well.

   After Jane got in touch with the part of her that blocks her sexuality and deadens her thighs, I suggested to her to personify the opposite. Instead of a morally judging self; she became her sensual pleasure-seeking self and danced to "Shaft" with an undulating pelvis.
7. Personifying symbolic process: Acting out dreams has long been a therapeutic method in Gestalt. Contrary to more traditional methods of analysis, Perls believed that every aspect of a dream, every character, every object in its environment are parts of the individual. By becoming these aspects, following the progression of the dream, each part conversing and contacting where appropriate with other aspects, self integration could more readily occur. Perls felt that the full gamut of an individual's conflictual behavior can manifest itself in one dream and that total therapy can be spent working with those symbols toward figure formation. (This belief is certainly in accord with the exploration of a dream of the individual described in the subsequent case study.)

*It is vitally important to make sure that the individual's breathing is in service to the natural flow and rhythm of the movement.

Other avenues for symbolic expression are also valuable such as the exploration of unconscious gesture or of significant objects or myths in the individual's external environment.

Role of the Therapist

Essentially it is the role of the therapist to assist and accompany the individual in his journey into heightened awareness of himself through the formulation and destruction of gestalts. She is a guide who suggests movement experiments which provide opportunities for action that facilitate an integration process. These creative environments stem from the clients' own images and behavior. Phrases, gestures, body attitudes can flower into rich metaphors for his life.

It is never the role of the therapist to make interpretations or to label behavior. She is a watch dog, assisting the individual to stay in the present pointing out to him when he talks "about" an emotion rather than feeling, uses "it" or "you" in lieu of "I" or curtails his experience by judgements, shoulds and expectations.

The therapist is her own instrument the Polsters claim, and that means to me that my body and its capacity to move, my feelings, my creative abilities, as well as my intuition, can all play a vital role in the creation of an experiment for growth.

It is vital for the therapist to trust herself and her own sensitivities. For example, in an initial session with Beth, described earlier, I suddenly became aware of an image: I pictured myself holding and rocking her telling her that I could care for her and accept her. She was talking "about" her existence which seemed to have no relationship to this fantasy; however, her tone of voice and body posturing told a different story. I took a risk at trusting my intuition and shared this fantasy with her. Beth cried fully for the first time. I touched her in a way that gave her support and care without stifling the expression of her grief and lonely longing. Giving support to an individual's expression and release is often a vital step toward risk taking. For example, by sensitizing Beth to a potential area of her own support: her back, through touching her spine periferally but contactfully, she was reacquainted with her own somatic support system, thus providing an inner base of strength from which to release feelings.

It should be clear in this last example that I do not always remain a passive observer. I feel it important that the individual see me as a living flowing person who is working with him toward his growth. I can feel confused, excited and jokingly happy and am able to share my experience when I feel it beneficial to his self-actualization. If we can experience contact between us, this process may aid in his evolution toward intrapersonal contact. If he can trust himself in our relationship, perhaps he can begin to better trust himself in the often painful risk-taking process of growth.

Clients often feel that the therapist has in some ways "caused" them to become more aware. In some instances it is as if the individual gives his own power for his therapy over to the therapist. Insuring that the individual takes full responsibility not only for his behavior but also for his growth is a vital premise in my work. I cannot "make" someone evolve; I have no magical powers (although I have been accused of such numerous times). I am a guide; and it is up to the client to choose to explore the suggested route toward integration.

And, finally I feel that training and experience in any therapeutic approach, however extensive, is meaningless if the dance therapist herself is not strongly rooted in her own self-actualization. She must know herself and have access to her own pain and fears. A client will often sense a therapist's personal discomfort, e.g., "If she doesn't trust and accept herself, how can I be acceptable?" Having experienced my own hidden gestalts and accepted the ongoing process of my growth, I can encourage and respectfully appreciate another's evolutionary process in all its depth and intensity.

I would like to share a quote by Polanyi (Polster, 1973) which speaks to this subject:

> . . . when we reach the point at which one man knows another, the knower (so) fully dwells in that which he knows . . . (that) . . . we arrive at the contemplation of a human being as a responsible person, and apply to him the same standards as we accept for ourselves, our knowledge of him has definitely lost the character of an observation and has become an encounter instead (P. 107).

Case Study

Sylvie was a married, 28 year-old woman of French origin who had come to the United States to get her doctorate in biochemistry. I first saw Sylvie in an ongoing dance therapy growth group that was composed primarily of students from the various universities in the city. She was referred to me via a counselor who had a fine intuitive sense of what dance therapy could offer certain individuals.

Sylvie was quietly composed in the group; she would join in interactional movement situations seemingly more out of an internal "should" than an integrated desire to explore with others. While some group members were able to involve their whole bodies in postural expressive sequences, Sylvie found this to be difficult. Her legs could move in a strong, direct, quick pattern, but the flow of dynamics would be blocked at her pelvis. Her breathing too was held and shallow. When the group would be involved in moving in free flow like "rag dolls," Sylvie's arms and legs would flow; however her head remained rigidly held to a bound torso. There was fear and sadness in her eyes while her mouth, jaw and neck remained tense.

Sylvie also chose not to extend her body into space. Her kinesphere* rarely evolved into intermediate space. Her upper torso stayed in a narrowed, hollowed empty position, while her pelvis rotated forward to accommodate this positioning of her chest.

It became also apparent that Sylvie shyed away from any movement experience that involved her taking a stand—feeling grounded in an affirmation of committment or presentation of self. She was continually observed moving in a twisting manner from one leg to another never balancing herself on both feet (Bernstein, 1975).**

Her favorite effort combination (body attitude) was that of indirectness and flow with a pre-effort of gentleness.*** She had a sensitive, evasive floating quality about her.

One evening the group was exploring in-depth unconscious authentic symbolic patterns. After awhile I suggested, as I often do in these explorations, to intensify the movement pattern in some way. I also asked them to allow a sound to come from that pattern through their breathing and finally, to begin to identify any feeling which may be associated as well as any environment which comes to mind.

**Kinesphere*—sphere-like projected space denoting an individual's comfortable or personal space. (Laban)

**This twisting shifting of weight pattern has been conceptualized as an "anal libidinal rhythm" by Dr. Judith Kestenberg (1965).

***Pre-effort: Involving the ability to cope with external forces of weight, space or time utilized in the motor expression of defense mechanisms. (Kestenberg, see Bernstein, 1975)

Sylvie, normally quiet and soft-spoken began evolving a deep gutteral sound. And finally, "get away, get away!" arose. Seated on the floor, she kicked out at the space in a rhythmic pattern, moving herself back "up against the wall." Her voice became higher pitched; fear of discovery and intensity had begun to cripple her expression.

It seemed difficult for Sylvie to share her experience verbally with the others in the group. However, the next morning, I received a call, "I've become aware of a lot of feelings I've been holding in. That was my mother I was kicking away last night. And I get these migraine headaches all the time, they just come on me and I can't do anything. I'd like to work with you individually. . . ."

In our first session together we evolved a contract. Sylvie wanted to stop having migraine headaches; they would "come on her" weekly and last for days. She would then take a prescribed drug which would make her regurgitate. She would have difficulty focusing, but feel that she had to go to the lab and work on her experiments. It became clear that Sylvie had made little or no time for her own leisure. It seemed also apparent that she felt that the migraines were something separate from herself and that they came upon her from the outside. They were clearly an unintegrated gestalt.

The suggestion that she gave herself migraines was quite a novel idea to Sylvie. I shared generally with her the concepts of self responsibility and self acceptance as well as some basic principles of Gestalt therapy—an approach which she herself elected to utilize. We then began the journey into the many unintegrated parts of Sylvie, through her bodily expression of symbols which brought her finally to a life freed of headaches.

The first experiment involved becoming more aware of and getting to know that very unacceptable so-called enemy: Sylvie's migraine.

As her personified villan, she curled up in a tight, bound ball on the floor. In a squeezed voice she snarled, "I am Sylvie's migraine; I have control over her; I let her relax for a little while, but she knows I'm in control. I'm tight and hard, and I hold on to her, and I won't let go."

I asked if she were in touch with the "under dog" or the part that is being held on to. She sat back in a limp state and responded to her villan in an ambivalent child-like voice, "Please let me go. Please leave me alone."

"No I won't. I make sure that you don't lose your head!"

It was clear that even when Sylvie stood on the chair looking down at the pillow representing her migraine, she was not yet ready to either send it away or integrate it.

Her migraine served a very real purpose for her—a purpose that she was not yet ready to accept. Gestalt formation had not occured as she was only beginning to explore and crystallize the figures from their long untapped background.

The next session upon my suggestion, Sylvie brought in a dream she had had that week. We worked several hours with it. She related the dream as follows:

"I am playing in the field with a group of people. A friend and I go to get something that is needed. He's a fun-loving easy going guy. He suddenly falls down and he injures his neck. He says everything is all right but I know it is really serious. I take him to my apartment and try to call the doctor who doesn't want to come. I go look at my friend and he can't lift up his head. I start seeing a skeleton through his skin, and I am afraid. I wake up."

Sylvie played all the parts moving from one to the other. Intensity developed when she, as the injured friend, began moving her head.

"I'm going to lose my head!" she screamed in terror. "I can't get up, my head's falling off! I feel so helpless." I suggested that this was not an unfamiliar feeling for her. She then flashed on her childhood and revealed that she had had polio which had at one point affected the muscles in her neck.

"Where are you now?" I asked her, and she set the stage for her childhood with her mother looking down at her.

As mother she moved about the room in a quick possessed manner. "Oh you're sick again," she retorted. "How can I take care of you, I'm worried about your father. I think we're going to be separated. Oh, I don't know what to do . . . I'll take care of you," she said with a martyrdom that would have made Joan of Arc look like a free-loader.

At the end of the session, Sylvie spoke of how the only time her mother would pay any attention to her was when she was ill; and when she did, it was always with a feeling that it was just asking too much of her. I suggested the sour milk image to her. "When your mother did comfort and nurture you, there was always a hidden agenda making her care, symbolic of milk, soured with mixed feelings. This seemed accurate to Sylvie and the image was to reappear in a later session when she came in touch with her need to vomit.*

Sylvie also spoke of her placating role in the family, how she tried to support and care for her mother who also would have bouts with migraines. She became the mother in a desparate attempt to provide a potential environment for her parents marital situation to reverse itself. It never happened.

A subsequent session, still working with the dream, was videotaped by both of us and subsequently viewed and mutually discussed to facilitate figural awareness. As in the past, being the injured friend, she got in touch with a primary experience.

She began to relive in the present, a past childhood incident: still getting over her polio, she was sent to her grandparents as her brother was ill; as two children were sick, it was too much for her mother to cope.

"I can't let grandma know I am sad and frightened," she said timorously, rocking herself in the corner, "or she'll tell mommy, and then mom won't want to care for me. I'm afraid daddy is going to go away . . . I don't want to be here. I feel all alone."

Sylvie's breathing quickened. A red flush of energy surged up her neck as the tension was released and her tears swelled forth. As suddenly as the sadness came, it departed. I encouraged her to allow herself to have her sadness, but it disappeared into the background. She stood up and ran about the room. "I have to hide. Someone's coming!" She ran over and pulled the plug of the record player from the socket. I suggested to her that perhaps she was running from her own feelings and me as representing someone who encourages her to explore them. I pointed out jokingly her "shutting off my power by pulling my plug," and we both laughed.

As she selected a record for us to dance to—a part of all our sessions, I reinforced the "okayness" of one's own individual rhythm for growth. This day we explored an experiment to increase her awareness of her center—the origin of strength and assertion. Sylvie selected the "Misa Luba" and as we moved about the room I asked her what she was feeling.

"I am a cat," she snarled subtlely. I noticed her pelvis still tilted forward and I helped her position it in a more central balanced grounded place.

*Note the connection of the reaction produced by the drug she took for her migraines.

"I am strong, I can lash out. I can grab food. . . ."

I suggested that we pull food down and bring it into our bodies in such a way as to reaffirm a vertical stance. Once affirmed, we moved into the horizontal-sagittal planes in an attempt to have her explore the use her hithertofore blocked strength, directed toward another.

"I'm pushing you away. Get away!" And for the first time Sylvie's upper torso bulged forward, transmitting strength from her pelvis into her shoulders and arms. (We were moving in a reciprocal push-pull pattern.) After the sequence, she smiled and looked at me with bright lively eyes. Having touched and lived her sad, weak, helpless self, she had begun to free her angry, strong, powerful self as well.

The following session, Sylvie brought in a card of Shakespeare's Ophelia she had received from a friend. She felt that it held a special meaning for her, but was unclear as to its significance. (See below)

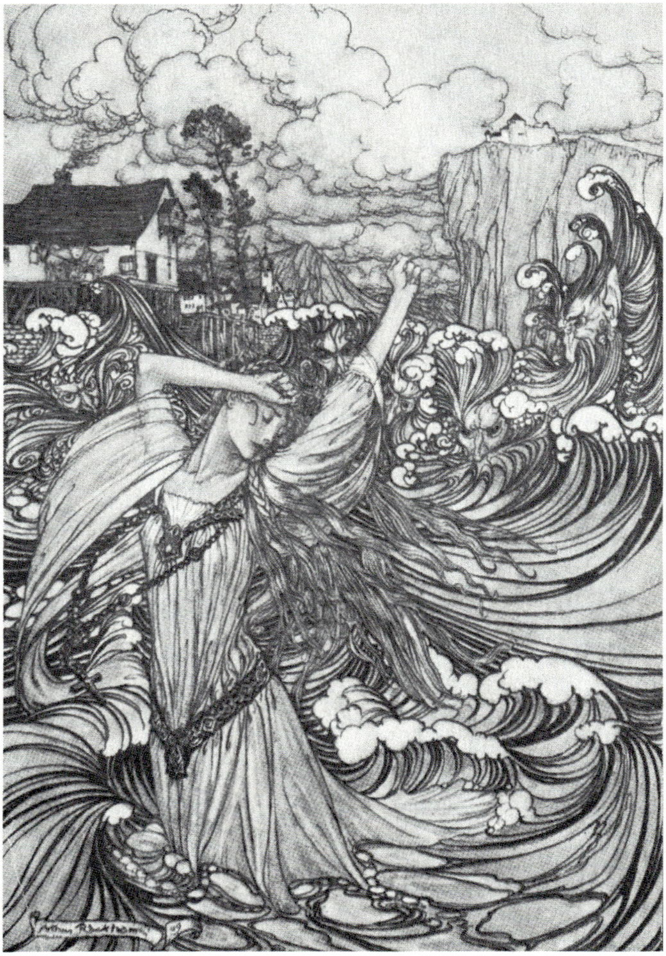

Sylvie became her Ophelia. She moved and writhed over the floor, every part of her flailing in extreme free flow. Once more I saw her neck vibrate with energy; this time it encompassed her whole torso. As she allowed her breathing to be in service of this pattern, her eyes opened wide with fear.

"I feel it from my belly. I feel frightened," and once more the experience began to subside. At this point I chose to reinforce her defense system rather than to attempt to create a new experiment which might bring her back into the feeling. I did this because I intuitively felt that it was important to help Sylvie become aware of how she blocks her experience, so that in the future she may have a choice as to when to utilize it and when to go with her feelings. Several times I had her close herself off: tensing her jaw and neck, cutting off her breathing, moving her body into an unaligned position, etc.; then release the armor and begin to experience; then close off again.

She gradually came to fully believe in her own control of herself and accept responsibility for her behavior and her choices.

"I've been giving myself migraines right after our sessions." "Good!" I said, "that means we're getting some place."

Sylvie then brought in a highly significant symbolic fantasy which emerged in a hallucination during her last migraine experience.

She related: "I started hearing a baby crying and I realized she was inside me. She was all locked up in the muscles in the back of my neck—right were my migraine is."

I suggested to her to live the fantasy as if it were happening now. As the child, Sylvie once more writhed on the floor. "Let me out! Let me out! I want to be free. . . ."

As the constricted migraine muscles, her body became rigidly tense. As she perched like a vulture, she said, "I'm not letting you out, if you come into Sylvie's brain you'll mix everything up!"

"I just want some love. I just want some time for me. I just want some care," responded the child. I suggested she stay with the feeling and repeat the phrase. She began to sob fully and deeply. Contact had occured.

As we talked through this intense experience, a lot of awareness began to come together for Sylvie. She realized that she never really allowed herself any time to relax; and that further, coming to see me was an indulgence that she had to punish herself for by giving herself a migraine—the controlling top dog which kept her child from having her needs met. Because she had locked up her child for so long—first with her martyred mother about whom she felt tremendous guilt asking for her time and care, and now with her own controlling parent who demands that she work constantly on her dissertation—she felt her needs and feelings to be omnipontent. "I feel if I ever really allow myself to be my child, I'll never want to get any work done." The issue of her feeling that she didn't have the right to take time for her child is manifested by: "How can I ask my mother for anything when she's suffering so much?" and "How can I take time out for myself when I've been given this scholarship to work?"

And finally, one of the more painful realizations for Sylvie became clear, her kinship with her mother. She too was playing the weak martyr who is deluged with migraines. However with this last awareness came a twinkling in her eyes: "I can choose to be this way or that."

At the end of the session, I suggested homework for her to do. Everyday, she had to spend at least one half hour indulging herself in a bath, doing some yoga relaxation, etc.

The next session Sylvie came in with two announcements: (1) she hadn't had a migraine and, (2) she felt a third person inside of her. "There's the controlling me, and the baby, and there's an aggressive me." With this phrase, she proceeded to move about the room with strong proud steps. "I argued back at my husband this week, and usually I withdraw and go numb." Still moving I put on a record and joined her exploring all the different possible forms that her new found strength could be expressed.

My association was that Sylvie's adult or ego had emerged and that this person is the rightful mediator between the child-id and the controlling parent-superego. If this part could truly be allowed figure formation, she would have no need of the migraines.

"Now you two work this thing out! Do you hear? Now look . . ." With two feet on th ground, Sylvie's so called "aggressive self" was assisting the other two parts of herself to come to some agreement. This "aggressive self" was a spontaneous figure formation which arrived for Sylvie via her inherent drive toward organismic self-regulation.

In subsequent sessions, Sylvie worked with her relationship with her mother. At one point I suggested to her to move in a bipolar symmetrical opening and closing pattern. When she found her own rhythm, I had her call for her mother. As she did so, her middle finger stiffened in anger. She became aware of a feeling of nausea and I suggested she find her own movement pattern for a symbolic regurgitation. The care from her mother had been soured by her sadness and Sylvie's bound-up unmet needs. She became aware that her relationships with all women had been soured as well as her acceptance of her own womanhood and her ability to be a good mother to herself.

In following sessions, she released and separated her angry feelings toward her mother in movement dramas involving her whole body. Gradually her tender feelings toward herself, the therapist and others began to emerge.

In one of her final hours—she shared a fairy tale that had special meaning for her:

"There was a dwarf in the castle that the King ordered to clean all the money in the dungeon in order to find the coin that was gold. Only then could he get out of prison."

She said that she didn't know why this story was so important to her until now. I suggested that she may have found her own gold of self-knowledge and was able to release herself from her own internal prison.

In Sylvie's last session, I suggested that she officially become her own therapist, she suggested the following work for the day:

"I'm becoming more aware of my pelvis. I can feel when I'm centered and I can feel my own potential to be strong. I'd like to explore that some more and make sure I'm breathing into my belly."

At the end of the session, she shared with me that she had felt herself giving herself a migraine the other day and so she "just walked around the apartment enjoying looking at old pictures" and it went away.

I told Sylvie to let me know if her migraines start up again—I haven't heard from her.

Bibliography

Bernstein, Penny. *Theory and Methods of Dance-Movement Therapy.* Second Edition, Dubuque, Iowa: Kendall/Hunt Publishing Co., 1975.

———, and Enzo Cafarelli. "An Electromyographical Validation of the Effort System of Notation," *Writings on Body Movement and Communication,* Vol. II, ADTA Pub., 1972.

———. "Range of Response as Seen Through a Developmental Progression," *What is Dance Therapy Really?* Govine and Smallwood, edts., ADTA Pub., 1973.
———. and Lawrence Bernstein, "A Conceptualization of Group Dance-Movement Therapy as a Ritual Process," *Writings on Body Movement and Communication,* Vol. III, ADTA Pub., 1973-4.
———. and Blaine Garson, "Pilot Study in the Use of Tension Flow System of Movement Notation in an Ongoing Study of Infants at Risk for Schizophrenic Disorders," *Dance Therapy—Depth and Dimension,* Delores Plunk, ed., ADTA, 1975.
———. "Tension Flor Rhythms: As a Developmental Diagnostic Tool Within the Theory of the Recapitulation of Ontogeny," *Dance Therapy—Dance and Dimension,* ADTA, 1975.
Rubin, Judith, Eleanor Irwin, and Penny Bernstein. "Play, Parenting, and the Arts," *Therapeutic Process Movement as Integration,* Penny Bernstein, ed., ADTA, 1975.
Bernstein, Penny. Editor, *Therapeutic Process Movement as Integration,* ADTA Pub., 1975.
———. "Dance-Movement Therapy," *Psychotherapy Handbook,* Richard Herink, ed., Jason Aronson, Inc., Pub. In process.
Fagen, J. and I. Shepherd. *Gestalt Therapy Now.* Palo Alto: Science and Behavior Books, Inc., 1970.
———. *What is Gestalt Therapy?* New York: Harper and Row, 1973.
Latner, Joel. *The Gestalt Therapy Book.* New York: Julian Press, Inc., 1973.
Lederman, J. *Anger and the Rocking Chair: Gestalt Awareness with Children.* New York: McGraw-Hill, 1969.
Naranjo, C. *Techniques of Gestalt Therapy.* SAT Press, 1973.
Perls, F *Ego, Hunger, and Aggression.* London: Alle and Anwin, 1947.
———, Hefferline, R. and Goodman, P. *Gestalt Therapy.* New York: Dell, 1965.
———. *Gestalt Therapy Verbatim.* California: Real Peoples Press, 1969.
Polster, I. and Polster, M. *Gestalt Therapy Integrated.* New York: Brunner-Brunner/Mazel, 1973.
Stevens, B. *Don't Push the River.* Layfayette, California: Real Peoples Press, 1969.
Stevens, J. *Awareness.* California: Real Peoples Press, 1971.
Watts, Alan. *Meditation.* Melbrae: Celestial Arts, 1974.

Presentations:

Bernstein, Penny and Leah Hall, "Cross Cultural Puberty Rituals and Jungian Dance Therapy: A Comparative Study," Presented at the 1977 ADTA International Conference. Available at Antioch-New England.
Bernstein, Penny and Wayne Coursol, "An Application of the Phenomenological Method in an Individual's Experience of a Jungian Dance Therapy Ritual Process," Presented at the 1977 ADTA International Conference. Available Antioch-New England.

Chapter 9

BODY EXPERIENCE WITHIN THE THERAPEUTIC PROCESS A PSYCHODYNAMIC ORIENTATION*

*Diane Fletcher, MA, DTR***

Genesis

In these last ten years, innumerable dimensions of body experience and ways of working with the body have evolved. I believe that it is necessary now that there are so many different body oriented therapies and techniques, that therapists using body experience as a therapeutic modality articulate with as much accuracy as possible the differences between and values of the various kinds of body and movement systems. I think it is important for each therapist to be developing basic understandings and concepts which relate body phenomena to the human organism as a whole and to develop a conceptual frame of reference which deals with the therapeutic treatment process. For this I feel it would be useful for dance therapy to be regarded within the broader context of psychotherapy of which it is a part and to draw from the legacy of psychotherapeutic knowledge. With this in mind, the purpose of this paper is to examine how I use body experience within a psychodynamic therapeutic process.

Further reading of this chapter will demonstrate that my approach and the phenomena arising from it have originated from the specific context, structure and clientele of my own practice and experience. Under different conditions such phenomena might not emerge and the work might not be directly applicable in the same way. My hope is that regardless of agreement or of similarity in theory or methodology, the reader will be stimulated to reconsider how he or she uses movement and body experience therapeutically and to question its relation to the total therapeutic process.

In stating how I have come to this approach, I must first state that I see myself as being in an ongoing process of learning. In no way do I feel that I have "arrived" or that the material in this chapter (which I wrote in 1974) is conclusive. However, as I look back of particular significance for me throughout this period of development is my own ongoing internal process of investigation. I believe this is essential for all dance therapists. I am talking about a continual, personal, detailed exploration of one's ever-changing experience of the body, movement and expressiveness in relation to the ever-changing sense of relation to others and life events. The more one can truly "know" oneself, the more one can also see and understand in others. I will forever be grateful to Mary Whitehouse for starting me out on this process. It was she who introduced

**Ms. Fletcher is in private practice in Los Angeles and is presently a Ph.D. candidate in clinical-social psychology at the Wright Institute, Los Angeles.

me to the internal world and to a way back to myself. From her came the first inspiration for "the search". From her I learned that there was such a thing as "listening" inside and as spending time with oneself. Though in many important ways I have pursued a different direction, I can feel Mary's influence on my work. One of the main influences from her is the emphasis on the very simple but difficult task of learning how to be able, in the moment, to locate and feel the nature of one's own experience inside one's body and to be able to follow that experience wherever it goes with conscious attention and respect, "letting it happen" without interferring. Mary's committment to the psychic experience which comes through working with the body and her committment to the consciousness of meaning that emerges in this process can be seen throughout my work.

Even before this my inclination for detailed study brought me to the mime Etienne Decroux in Paris. It was Decroux who taught Marcel Marceau. Six months of extensive study with Decroux primed me to pay minute attention to the articulation of the body.

In relation to self knowledge, a lengthy psychoanalysis has contributed greatly. Years have been spent working within myself trying to grasp at both the intuitive and intellectual level; the relation of my bodily experiences to my sense of self. I personally felt the need to be able to really utilize the body experiences for deep internal change. My own work is a reflection of that pursuit. However input from the outside was also essential. Extensive and long-term psychoanalytically oriented supervision with Dr. Stephen Rush and a good deal of reading in various areas of psychodynamic theory and practice, have made this work possible. Otherwise, I would have been "stuck" just with my own process.

Though the material in this chapter centers on my individual work with clients, I have been influenced by my expereinces as a dance therapist at St. Elizabeth's Hospital, Washington, D.C. where Marian Chace evolved her group work in dance therapy. It is, of course, impossible to try to summarize the many understandings I gained there, but certainly one of the most powerful ideas which I have continued to explore is that of group process, as it occurs both verbally and non-verbally. Though the context of group process is obviously different from that of individual work, there are some similarities in the task. The therapist must try to grasp what is going on at a given moment and to relate to that in a meaningful way.

In most of the experiences I mentioned there is a common theme. How does one learn to recognize that which is obvious and essential but often unobserved? Often that which is really the most essential, the most real and significant goes unnoticed. A primary value is placed on the ongoing search for truth and reality and on the meaningful development of inner psychic life and of interpersonal relations, all of which are viewed in the context of the ongoing fabric of experience. These basic observations are not new at all; in fact, they may be so familiar that they seem deceptively unimportant. The significance is "right there" on the surface in the experience, if one can only learn to "see" it.

The special emphasis given above to the overall process is not meant to overshadow the importance of detailed and disciplined learning in specific areas of knowledge. Of special importance for me was my graduate work at U.C.L.A. with Dr. Alma Hawkins who started me thinking and conceptualizing and with Dr. Valerie Hunt whose understanding of movement and whose method of movement observation based on Laban's work has been of much use to me. Along the way a substantial period of meditation as well as the use of imagery developed by Ira Progoff have added considerable dimension. A deeper and more detailed understanding of the structure of the body began when I audited the training program for Structural Integration developed by

Ida P. Rolf. Here I began to "see" and understand the body in a new way. This process, of course, has continued.

Of just as much importance in developing my present approach is the work itself which evolves as one is doing it. I am, of course, forever being taught by my clients. Clearly, the kind of clientele I have worked with has influenced my work considerably.

Theoretical Model

Concepts

Relationship of Physical and Mental Modes

Our Western culture distinguished, at least to some degree, between what is psychical, mental or spiritual and what is tangible, material or physical. The following relations between mental and physical modes are often observed. Events which are represented mentally are functionally and/or symbolically related to physical expressions and internal bodily events. Physical and mental modes link up, interact and trigger each other. This is the basis of psychosomatic medicine. The expressions of the various physical and mental modes reflect or suggest the identity and organization of the total personality. This is the basis of the projective psychological testing. (Rush, 1973) It may seem redundant to reiterate these obvious facts which are seen, though may be difficult to explain, but their significance as the theoretical underpinnings of a working therapeutic process must not be minimized. It is in working with these different modes and the complicated ways in which they interact that the way to the whole person and the underlying schemata or dynamics by which the personality is organized can be found.

By the term physical mode, I am referring to both the actual, tangible physical events and to their psychical components as they are represented and appear in conscious, preconscious or unconscious functioning. In more specific terms, this is to say that even though I may be involved with the fact of a particular gesture which I see the client doing, I am also paying close attention to the client's and my psychological experience of it.

I am assigning the term mental mode to the more psychical aspects of our functioning. This includes such psychical phenomena as image, imagination, dream, symbol formation, memory, intuition, intention, will, thought, and language. Of course, in the psychical mode, time and space are highly fluctuating and variable. Psychically the range of possible experiences are infinite. Trying to understand the differences between the mental and physical modes of functioning applies in a very immediate way to the dance therapist, for she is always working with the whole person even though the physical experience is given special emphasis. She cannot afford to forget that there is a whole psychical world of meaning around those physical events with which she might be working. Nor can she afford to forget that much of this psychical world is not available through the physical mode by itself. The relation of the mental mode to the physical must not be taken for granted. I believe that anyone working psychotherapeutically with the body must be careful of making simple mind/body equations, that is, assuming that what happens in a physical mode also happens in an equivalent way in the structure of the human psyche. This is only sometimes the case. Sometimes there are direct equivalencies, for instance in which a viscera or motor behavior, often referred to as a symptom, will resonate as a physical expression of a particular perception, thought or feeling. Or, sometimes a gesture, or sensation will be an exact replication of one detail in a memory which is being re-enacted. However, just as frequently the different physical expressions do not have a direct equivalent relation to a given perception, thought or feeling. The physical expression may be a response or reaction to the initial feeling; it may be a defense against the feeling or a transformation of it.

Sensation

Research indicates that with every thought, perception, or bit of emotion, there is some specific neuromuscular pattern in the smooth or striated muscle. (Jacobson, 1967) This motor activity is usually unobserved, but if desired it is available to conscious perception as bodily sensation. Physical sensation can be felt in many ways: motor or visceral sensations, postural tension, kinesthetic and joint sensations which contribute to awareness of shape, size, position and location in space; sensations of the breathing apparatus; and of various qualities of motion, amount of effort, and qualities of stillness and constriction.

For instance, at a given moment if I make an action, there will be a whole pattern of sensations which report to me the attitude and quality of that behavior in relation to the muscular innervation involved. Is the attitude enthusiastic, hanging back, heavy, slow and depressed, frantic, lingering, dawdling or bored? All of this would be represented in sensations arising from the posture, gait, gestures, quality of motion, tension, etc. These subliminal sensations can be utilized as internal information to help understand what is felt. Ideally, the information is integrated as a feeling of self. In everyday experience the pieces and bits of experience in terms of separate sensations are not usually noted, but the internal signaling and feedback is still going on in the background as part of our personal experience and identity. Thus, all mental events involve some level of neuromuscular innervation. This physical innervation is signaling back to the psychic part of our functioning as sensation. Providing it is not disrupted, this is an ongoing process of internal self-recognition, feedback and connection between physical and mental modes of experience. Much of this chapter has to do with the ways in which this connection is furthered or disrupted.

Sensation then, involves both the physical and mental mode. It is the means by which a neuromuscular event is registered psychically. Thus it is an important internal system of communication or language. Sensation is one of the body's ways of telling us what's happening inside in relation to oneself, to others and events. For instance, in young children, the person or object from whom they get what they want feels 'good' to them, and the person or object from whom they do not get what they want feels to them to be 'bad'. (Isaacs, 1933) The designation "good" and "bad" refer to the gratified or frustrated inner feelings of the child projected onto the object. The pleasureful or negative sensations we have in relation to the other is one of the first ways a meaningful evaluation and response to the objects in our world is construed. Jacobson (1967) indicated this in his conception of emotions, which views the specific neuromuscular patterns and sensations as the means by which man apprehends and evaluates reality. As internal signals, sensations are a means internally of representing oneself to oneself both in relation to the perceived external world and in relation to the internally represented world.

Body Schemata

In the previous paragraphs, I have discussed how internal events are represented as sensations. Research also indicates that the body is mentally represented to the person as image—body image. (Schilder, 1950) The mental images by which the body is represented are rich and varied. They may be fragmentary or complete; they represent all aspects of the body, against which the momentary body information is filtered, compared and organized.

Sometimes, due to various circumstances and internal phantasies, certain basic body schemata are prevented from being formed or are formed in a distorted way. This distorts the capacity to organize present incoming information. If for instance, a person has a distorted schema regarding his skin as the means by which he is physically enveloped as the boundary between self and not self, a deep confusion as to identity, boundaries, self-differentiation and basic safety may ensue.

The basic composite body image or scheme constitutes the means by which a perceptual constant is formed as a part of the person's self image. It provides a constant for the moment to moment images of the body which are continually changing, forming, reforming, being torn down, fragmenting, multiplying and superimposing themselves on the next image. The moment to moment representations of the body do not change the more constant body scheme. However traumatic, intense or especially integrated body experiences can alter the organization of the basic body scheme. This is what I understand dance therapists to mean when they speak of changing the body image.

Object-Relations

It is important to recognize that the meaning of the motor patterns is not explicitly expressed by body language or by the internal language of sensation and body image. What the gestures, images and sensations are referring to, what they are "all about" must be interpreted. For there to be meaning the actions and impulses must be related to their object. Meaning derives from a relationship between subject and object. The object may be an internally represented one or an externally perceived one, usually a combination of the two.

Sometimes the objects toward which one's actions intend is directly perceived and related to in the external world. However often the implied object and related associations is only unconsciously represented. One lashes out *at,* yearns *for,* withdraws *from,* hungers *for,* thinks *about,* and feels *toward* "something"; though one may not know what that something is. In daily life, one is frequently lacking the conscious thought which would express the whole intention or meaning. The body work can often help bring to conscious foreground the subjective impulse toward action. However, the work is incomplete until the object and the relation to the object is brought out. Much of the work of therapy has to do with uncovering and articulating this area of meaning, that is—the relations between the many parts of the self with their conflicting impulses to their many objects.

It is important to remember that these relations between the subject and object occur psychically as well as externally. Often it is discovered how one has been trying to interact with the external world, but that the interactions have very little to do with that world. Rather, it is discovered that one is relating to an illusion of the real world and that was based on an internal psychic construction. Locating and working with these constructions or schemata is an essential part of therapy. I am referring here to the unconscious internal representation of a person's early relationships to the important people and events in his life. These early representations form many of the basic ideas and expectations about oneself, significant others and one's relationship to them, and they become the basis of patterns which are often acted out throughout life.

> The theory of *psychic structure* evolved from Melanie Klein's clinical findings was to the effect that it consisted of phantasied or imaginary ego-object relationships which had become persistent, almost permanent, organizational features of the deeper psychic life. (Guntrip, 1961, p. 219)

Thanks to the clinical research of Melanie Klein (see reference list), a student of Freud's, we have a clearer understanding of how the intra-psychic structure is organized according to these early object-relations. In her theory of psychic structure she outlines the relation of somatic impulses to objects. She went back to Freud's concept of instinct and of instincts represented in the psychic life by mental representatives. Unconscious phantasy is viewed as the mental representative of impulses. The unconscious phantasy life is viewed on a continuum of impulses of loving libidinal desires toward the object and of aggressive death wishes to destory or get rid of the object. She emphasized that phantasy is first a non-verbal experience that starts as a somatic experience, then becomes visual and then more like verbal forms, narrative in nature. Explicit in Klein's view is that there are object-relations from the start and that instincts are object-seeking. It is generally expected that the rudimentary, infantile or primitive object-relations continue to exist in unconscious phantasy and that they continue to exert their influence even though they are repressed in the normal adult.

The detailed way in which one reconstructs and manifests the internal world is not just mental in terms of perception, image or thought; it is also physical. As will be recalled, all mental activity is reflected in the body in terms of some motor or visceral activity. The body as well as the psyche acts out the object-relations of unconscious phantasy. Reich (1933) speaks of the past as being embodied in the form of character attitude or character armor. In psychodynamically oriented dance-movement therapy the work is to find how these internal patterns manifest themselves and interact with the objects in the present. This is one reason why working with the transference reactions and projections onto the therapist is so valuable. Here the client vividly experiences over and over how he is repetitiously reconstructing and reliving one version after another of his psychic structure with the therapist in the transference reactions and projections. The immediacy of this experience has "greater force of conviction" which is unlikely to be forgotten. (Freud, 1940) The release and reliving of memory and unconscious phantasy which often comes up in body work is valuable, but ultimately it must be correlated in actual detail with the manner in which it is acted out in the transference and daily life.

To summarize, then, whether referring to infantile or adult levels of organization, I am discussing the linkage and interaction between physical and mental modes as they occur continually in a person's internal and external object-relations and thus in the psychic structure. Meanings are represented at both conscious and unconscious levels by a cross-referencing of the physical and mental modes. Sensations, impulses and intentions toward action, functional movements, expressive motion, body images, images, etc., are cross-referenced in relation to present perceptions of internal and external objects. From infancy onward these experiences are linked together through unconscious phantasy into schematic units of meaning (psychic reality) which effect moment to moment experiencing. (Isaacs,* 1943) Because of this inherent link each mode triggers the other and refers to the deeper meaning and dynamics by which the whole personality is organized. Generally the deeper meanings are not explicitly represented to consciousness as complete understandings. By paying attention to the bits and pieces of experience as they present themselves to awareness through dynamic association, the deeper meanings will begin to become more evident and available to conscious experience, integration and change. The body expressions, sensations, postures, images or ideas may bring forward a clarifying dream, a burst of feeling or

*Isaacs was a student of and collaborator with Klein. Her work "The Nature and Function of Phantasy" is very relevant to dance therapists.

a memory of particular event. Thus the very process of focusing on body experience tends to draw out the psychological content and the dynamic organization to which the body experiences are linked. Such is the basis of the use of body experience as a means toward intrapsychic reorganization.

Methods of Identification—Four Aspects of Experience

At this point it must be asked how these theories are pertinent to actual therapeutic practice. How is identifying and working with these so-called psychodynamics and their physical and mental expressions carried out?

Obviously the kind of material discussed in this last theoretical section must emerge in the client's ongoing process and experience within the context of the therapeutic relationship. This includes, of course, the client's evolving experience of inner "psychic reality", in relation to his daily living and in relation to me. In terms of the ongoing therapeutic process, I am particularly interested in four aspects of experience; subjective experiencing; identifying and reflecting on the content of the experience; identifying the action and/or mechanism; and linking. These four aspects also occur to some degree at all times in the course of ordinary daily experience.

Just to survive, one must be able to some degree, to experience oneself in the world and in relation to each other (subjective experiencing). One must be able to cognitively recognize and identify those experiences and to some degree determine their reality and meaning (identifying and reflecting on the content of experience). One must be able to see the consequences of one's actions and to know that to some degree the quality of living a feeling is contingent on the way one creates and searches out one's own experience (identifying the action and/or mechanism). And, one must somehow be able to link all of these aspects together in an organized way as to integrate some degree of meaning and purpose out of the experience (linking). Since these four aspects are involved in the everyday moment to moment organization of experience it is not surprising to find them essential in therapy. The use of body experience within the therapeutic process will be seen within the context of these four aspects. Of course all four of these aspects occur simultaneously or in varying sequences and combinations. Dividing these aspects of experience into four categories is a device for sake of discussion. Such a division does not really occur in the actual process.

Subjective Experiencing

By "experiencing", I am referring to the immediacy of one's own perception of self and to the quality of being. This refers to the "being person" as opposed to the "doing person". At a given moment, what is one's experience of one's self, how does one feel inside? The experience might be non-specific, a feeling, state or mood. It could be localized in a particular place or be in a very global undifferentiated sense of oneself. Being able to experience fully in personal relation to one's sense of identity is sustaining and enriching to the total personality.

By "experiencing", I mean the subjective and receptive capacity of allowing into consciouness both sensory data from the external world and internal perceptions such as sensation, image, fantasy and thought. This involves the capacity to allow the sensory and perceptual elements of experience to be felt as fully as possible.

In an experience it is important to discover where a sense of the self or personal identity is located and with what among the many possible elements of experience does the client identify.

Here, I am referring to the feeling of presence or absence of a subjective sense of "me", "myself" and how it links up to the element of experience.

Distortions in the experience of oneself are not uncommon. Even in so-called neurotics it is not uncommon to find symptoms that are often labeled as psychotic, for instance when parts of the self or of the perceptual apparatus are split off from the sense of self and then projected outside onto some object, or when parts of the perceptual apparatus itself are internally disrupted so as to prevent the perception and experience of a too painful reality. (Bion, 1957) These mechanisms are unconscious and therefore not usually experienced, but they may cause great anxiety and an experiece of losing oneself due to the seeming disappearance of a necessary part of self or function. For instance, vision may blurr or there may be difficulty in hearing and linking up words in a meaningful way. Awareness itself and a sense of the self may be experienced as splitting, fragmenting, sinking or swooning. Body parts may feel as if they are disappearing, growing numb, or disconnected. The capacity for sensation and therefore an essential part of self recognition may be muted, numbed or blanked out.

In therapy, the capacity for experiencing is enriched and intensified as new experiences are "discovered" or brought to consciousness by the process of association as originally developed by Freud. (Freud, 1940) In this process both physical and mental elements of experience are brought into association with each other and into relation with the self. There is an inner dialogue. When elements of experience are noted, questions are asked; and answers from the preconscious aspects of the personality emerge. The question asking function of the therapist facilitates this inner dialogue and the capacity to take council with oneself (Abraham, 1974). Association, as applied to body experience, means allowing the bits of sensation, motion, impulses, body images, etc., to "come up" to consciousness, to be felt and to be brought into meaningful relation to the subjective sense of self or identity and to the world.

It is often here through spontaneous association of one bit of experience to another that larger meaningful patterns emerge. Gradually through this process the deeper underlying schemata by which the personality is organized come to the surface of consciousness. The process of association taps into the dynamic organization and enables previously unconscious material to emerge and be experienced both physically and psychically, thus fostering the process of intra-psychic reorganization.

Initially, it may require some patience and time to learn how to associate, attend to, and follow the spontaneous unfolding of inner experience. For some people, just feeling the tangible actuality of sensation, any sensation, is quite a new and sometimes frightening experience. As the capacity to "pay attention" and focus on subjective experience develops, the sense of personal identity is heightened. The link between mental content, emotion and sensation is often vividly felt. Experience becomes substantial, that is tangibly defined in the musculature and viscera and articulated in image, thought, memory and feeling. If the capacity to experience is blocked, as it frequently is by physical tension, there may be a psychological sense of emptiness, void, numbness or apprehension; there may be a feeling of something dead or missing.

Identifying and Reflecting on the Content

By identifying and reflecting on the content I mean paying specific conscious attention to, recognizing the actual details of what is going on in an experience and making those details the object of inquiry and reflection. In this way one's subjective experiences become the object of thought. This is necessary for a basic level of mastery. By mastery I mean the capacity to control and determine the basic direction in one's life and daily living. Such a level of functioning requires that one must be able to recongize, attent to and think about what is happening. The different parts of an experience must be differentiated. This aspect of processing an experience calls for the observing, containing and reflective capacities of the ego. In this process perceptions arising from internal cues and reactions are differentiated from external circumstances. (Freud, 1933) Present information is correlated with other knowledge from past experience. By these means, a given situation is estimated and evaluated in terms of internal motives, cues and external requirements. Other possibilities can be devised in relation to priorities and goals. Such actions are required for autonomous functioning. They are involved in the functioning of the "reality principle" of the ego as outlined by Freud, (1940). The ego's capacity of reality testing brings intellect, reason and reflection together with experience. In this way the objective and subjective aspects of the self are integrated. Bit by bit experiences can be broken down into observeable, nameable events and reorganized in relation to the present context. It is this processing of information and new experience that helps to bring about a reorganization of the existing patterns. This is where verbalization becomes so important; observing, identifying, locating and naming are all tools of mastery. One does not need to be dominated by an over-subjective orientation in which experiences are felt to be impinging and overwhelming. Experience can be broken down into useful bits to be digested, assimilated, organized and integrated.

Identifying the Actions and/or Mechanism

To change ones life and stop repetitive patterns is needed more than the capacity to subjectively experience, identify and reflect on these patterns. One needs to be able to do something about them. One needs to be able to get a "handle" on them. Such a "handle" is gained when one learns to identify and control the actions and/or mechanisms by which experience is created, altered or destroyed. How personal meaning and reality are actively constructed, how perceptions, reactions, feeings, thoughts, phantasies and behaviors from moment to moment are sought, selected and created, must be examined. This aspect of experience refers to the self as the *doer.* Identifying the physical actions and psychological mechanisms a person uses to make an experience happen or not happen relocates the responsibility and control back inside that person so that events do not any more "just happen".

Many of the mechanisms by which one creates experience are physical. The way in which one uses his body can often change how one feels. This is the "magic" of the body. By manipulating body experience, one can often physically and/or emotionally reconstitute oneself to some degree, at least for the moment.

This capacity to alter immediate experience is a basic survival mechanism learned from infancy on. It involves first learning how to distinguish "good" from "bad" and then learning how to organize oneself accordingly. Freud rightfully said that "the ego is first and foremost a body ego". (Freud 1927) As outlined in his pleasure pain principle, some sensations and body experiences are pleasurable and one seeks to further them. Others are unpleasant or painful and one works to get rid of them. (Freud, 1940) This is done in various ways, and usually one is not conscious of what it means that one is seeking certain pleasurable experience and avoiding unpleasant ones. If the experience threatens to be dangerous or "bad" a person just tries immediately to fix it by getting rid of the "bad" feeling in some way or another.

Psychoanalyst Rado (1969) referred to this as "riddance behavior". He quotes Darwin on this subject, describing how aninals will often shake a hurt body part as if to shake off the cause. He claims how many behaviors such as repression which are usually classified as defense mechanisms can be seen as riddance behaviors, for they have as their aim the riddance (rid-dance) of some threatening thought, emotion or experience. Freud (1933) outlines many psychic defense mechanisms which are employed to eliminate any threatening or overwhelming awareness to the total personality.

There are countless examples in our daily lives of movement or alterations in tension as riddance behavior. Many people for instance deal with depression by becoming very active doing almost anything so as not to feel what might be a heavy, scary, immobile or death-like feeling that comes on when they sit still. Disturbed persons who must exert a great deal of effort trying to control their rages and fears, have extremely distorted and tense bodies, bodies which in themselves are felt as a threat; for at any moment the intense feelings might break through on a physical level. They may try to dissociate from their bodies so as not to experience the bombardment of sensations and associated physical and psychic pain. Creating alterations in muscle tone through tension and flaccidity is one of the major motor defense mechanisms (Fletcher, 1974).

It is noteworthy that most of the time a person does not even know physical action is being taken or body sensation is being modified in some way in order to get out of a threatening or anxious state. Such moods or states often come on subtly—a flash of an image, a fragment of a thought, a glimpse of a threatening fantasy, a twinge of a frightening sensation, some bit of motion or posture that reminds one of something threatening but unknown. The quick and subtle body action to get rid of the threatening moment usually happens subliminally. Much of the neurotic's life is spent getting rid of real, remembered or imagined threats in such a way. Because these mechanisms occur out of awareness, they are therefore out of conscious control. However with awareness and understanding, many of these defensive motor mechanisms can potentially be brought under more conscious control and the underlying feelings can thereby be more readily tapped.

Therapeutic Implication of Riddance Behavior as a Motor Defense

The natural survival function of riddance behavior has implications for dance therapists. It is important to be alert to the differences between useful or counter-therapeutic uses of riddance behavior. In daily living, getting rid of bad feelings and anxiety is a natural, though often fatiguing function. Obviously, the less energy we have to spend on defending ourselves by getting rid of our expereinces, the more we might have to develop for creative living. However, in therapy we must examine the implications of such behavior. It might feel better to "dance out" the threatening feelings and to make oneself "feel better", at least temporarily; however by doing just this the opportunity to really discover what those unbearable thoughts and feelings are is passed by. If in therapy, the relief of discharging feelings and thoughts is consistantly sought before the difficult feelings have been experienced and identified, then the opportunity for change that comes from working through the threatening experience has been aborted. Often this results in the repetitive attempt to rid oneself of the ever returning feelings. With this in mind it is very important to determine whether the body is used as a defense against whatever experience might be emerging at the time or whether the body experience furthers it.

There are times of course when particular riddance behaviors may be valuable in momentarily relieving a person, thereby reducing enough intensity and anxiety to gain control. The element of control from within and self mastery in the world is always of prime consideration. It is a fundamental need to be in at least some control of one's experience, to be able to preserve the "good" and get rid of the "bad". I am underscoring this obvious fact since it seems to have become popular to consider control as "bad" and defensive, and to consider defenses as "bad". It seems to me that without the feeling that we can regulate our experiences to at least some degree, we will not feel safe enough to be able to "open up" to new experiences.

Particularly with more disturbed persons, a very legitimate use of dance therapy is in helping the client take responsibility for his emotional condition, helping him find a constructive means of discharging the built up tensions of negative emotion by rechanneling it into acceptable action. This use of body expereince is reconstitutional. Indeed there are often times when one cannot reach what is causing the upsetting experience in time to defuse it, and by that time there is already a physical build up of excitation in the muscles which must be dealt with. But I think we must make the distinction between temporarily discharging the physical excitations and the assumption that discharge will get rid of or "release" the person in any lasting way. I do not believe that it can. On the other hand, there are other occasions where discharge, if accompanied by emotion, thought and memory in the context of a present experience, can then be used toward psychic reorganization and structural change.

Linking

By linking, I am referring to the process by which the elements of experience are internally connected in meaningful association with each other and organized in a uniquely coherent way. (Saul, 1972) The importance of linking has already been alluded to some degree in the conceptual section. From infancy onward, a person comes to know the self and world by linking up aspects of experience into meaningful schemata. Different sensory modalities and physical and mental elements of experience must be linked in order to "know something." Internal and external cues must be organized and differentiated. Basic life experiences must be integrated in order to form a coherent representation of the self and the world. Without this, one could not navigate.

I believe that extreme alterations in muscle tone in the form of tension and flaccidity is one of the basic methods by which one interferes with the linking process. Tension and flaccidity interfere with the internal proprioceptive feedback system which is necessary in order to process information. I have been working on this in relation to schizophrenia and am studying this motor defense mechanism in newborns as a basic defense when regulatory difficulties occur within the newborn and/or when the mother and newborn interaction is not able to meet the regulatory needs of the newborn. I think this is an important area of investigation for dance therapists.

Perhaps it is a familiar experience for those who work with very disturbed persons to come upon a situation in which a patient didn't know that the burning sensation in his body just bfore he impulsively hit someone was aggressive rage. In such a case, the sensations were not linked to a psychological awareness of rage. Had they been so linked, the sensation might have been identified by the patient as some form of emotion, intentful action, or destructive imagery in relation to the object. If any of these bits of experience had been associated in the patient's awareness there might have been the possibility of control. A more common example is that of having a tight feeling in the throat and not realizing that it is a sign of some emotion, perhaps needing a cry, or of not knowing about what one wants to cry.

Any interference with this linking would serve to disrupt the integrative process by which one's experiential and perceptual, moment to moment reality is created. Bion, (1957) has pointed out a potent defense mechanism which occurs frequently in psychotics and more subtly in others; he shows that if reality is too painful and/or overwhelming the perceptual apparatus and linking capacity by which that reality is constructed and brought into consciousness may be psychically attacked. The internal destruction of these links which connect the various internal signals associations and sensory impressions result in the destruction or alteration of the perception of reality.

There are many ways of disturbing, altering or destroying some element or linkage in the experience. A sensation may be split off from its emotional context; an image or idea may be left so partial as to be experienced as bland, useless, meaningless or disturbing. By ridding the self or certain elements of experience the total configuration in which one element is linked to another is changed and the threatening nature of the original experience is avoided.

What has been discussed here is rudimentary—the linking up of the experiencing, observing, doing and integrating aspects of the self into an organized whole person. With this comes the beginnings of self-knowledge and choice.

Therapeutic Process

Therapeutic Uses of Body Experience

From this material a number of observations concerning the various therapeutic uses of body experience can be drawn. I find that most body oriented techniques can be placed in one or more of these five categories: (1) discovering of new experience; (2) coping through reconstitution; (3) physical restructuring; (4) interpersonal communication; and (5) intra-psychic reorganization through insight into meaning. Though each category deserves extensive discussion, I hope it will be evident that even though most techniques overlap and involve more than one category, the emphasis does indeed make a difference and that each emphasis offers different benefits and has different drawbacks according to the specific needs of the individual.

The first category is that of *discovery.* By this, I am referring to having new experiences, broadening and enriching the range of movement qualities, the repertoire of actions, sensations and awareness. Often this must occur at a very basic level—learning about body parts, discovering what it feels like to have sensations at all, or in certain places, becoming aware that the body can move in different ways and that, for instance, it doesn't break. If there is no new experience at some level nothing will be learned. Some new dimension, sometimes that of awareness, or of different sensory perception must be found in even the most repetitive experience for there to be change.

Body work that is *reconstitutional* is based on the fact that the body can be worked with in order to assist a person to feel better. Many times such a process is referred to as "release" or "discharge." There is a common assumption that if one "expresses" i.e. discharges the negative feelings he will "get them out" and "feel better." Expression as discharge for the purpose of riddance in contrast to expression as communication to assist in the reorganization of experience, is a common means of coping. Certain movements, body positions, and free flow patterns such as udulation and swings or explosive patterns such as hitting and kicking often used in dance therapy assist a person in "letting go" and feeling better, in "getting rid" of anxiety or "bad" feelings.

Relaxation, and other forms of anxiety reduction are also often used before verbal therapy to facilitate a freer response.

In reconstitutional work, there may be educational aims beyond that of momentary relief. The goals may be to teach a person how to take care of himself, how to take charge of his condition, handle his anxiety and emotions and to help himself feel better. Such a process may be depicted as being a parent to oneself. Learning how to recognize and let go of tensions, to relieve oneself of bodily discomfort and to enjoy the pleasures of free spontaneous movement are significant human capacities which many people in contemporary society have not developed. For many persons, especially hospital patients, this kind of learning is very beneficial.

There are some drawbacks however. I have already noted that constantly trying to get rid of bad body feelings does not always help or solve the problems. Also when release techniques are applied, especially out of context, charged emotional material or disturbing memories and thoughts may come too abruptly to consciousness or defense mechanisms may be broken with the possible result of disorganizing the personality. Some of these techniques are quite powerful and could be damaging to persons who do not have strong, healthy defenses. Often the release of material requires therapeutic work in order for it to be utilized and integrated. Whether or not the leader works verbally with the material or makes a referral depends on the therapeutic or non-therapeutic nature of the contract and on the whether the dance therapy is being used as a primary or adjunctive therapy.

The third category is that of *restructuring* with the goal of physically restructuring the body so that the movement and postural organization of the body is not just reconstituted, it is actually physically restructured at a neuromuscular level. Structural Integration originated by Ida P. Rolf is an example of such work. There are time when restructuring is extremely valuable, but there are other times when such work is too advanced and unable to be utilized because the awareness of the body is so undeveloped and/or disturbance is so great that alignment is almost immediately redistorted. I might add that such systems often have the effect of relieving tension, of reconstitution, and sometimes of assisting intra-psychic change.

The fourth category, that of *interpersonal communication* involves the use of body experience for the purpose of relating to another. The movement itself or pure body aspects of the experience are not so important. What counts is the body expression as communication, as human exchange and contact. This work, orginally developed by Marian Chace, is the basis of a good deal of group work with hospitalized patients, especially non-verbal schizophrenics. Here, the body functions as a primary mode of communication and socialization. The focus is on interpersonal experience. Reconstitutional experiences are likely to occur in such a group but the emphasis is on the group dynamic and interpersonal feelings and interactions. Movement operates as a medium, like language, by which interpersonal skills and relations can be developed and an initial feeling of self through relating to others can be found.

In the fifth category, that of *intra-psychic reorganization through insight into meaning,* body experience is used as a tool to bring pre-verbal and undifferentiated experiences up to the level of conscious feeling, insight and thought. Newly discovered body experiences such as sensation, motion, posture, gesture and tension, etc., are a means of direct information and knowledge of the inner self. By being consciously experienced and verbalized, they are brought into association with thought, memory and intention; that is, meaning is realized. The emphasis here is on intra-psychic reorganization and a coherent, integrated connection between mental and physical processes.

When emotion is released within a meaningful context, new perceptions, ideas, memories or images emerge into consciousness and become available to be fed back to consciousness for further insight and integration. Often when there is a discovery of a new experience, emotion and insight emerge together and are then followed by a feeling of relief which comes with the new integration.

The distinctions I am trying to make in these catgories are intended as an attempt to clarify the uses of body experience. Clearly, the task of the therapist is to try to identify under what conditions, and for what purposes which uses of body experience are effective and which are counter-therapeutic.

Treatment Process—General Description

Many important aspects of the treatment process have been taken up throughout the chapter in the context of other concepts. Just to summarize, I would like to stress that fundamental psychodynamic processes are utilized. This includes continually working with the transference reactions and projections as they emerge in the ongoing client-therapist relationship. In this context, individual experience is understood from an object-relations point of view. The verbal and movement process of association is considered essential in that it taps in to the dynamic organization and enables previously unconscious material to emerge and be expressed both physically and psychically, thus fostering the process of intra-psychic reorganization. The treatment process also involves dealing with resistances and defenses. It involves repeatedly working through the distorted patterns and conflicts. Over and over, in different versions, conflict and tension are restated, encountered and mastered. This process occurs from month to month, session to session and during the course of the hour. Throughout this process, the client's trust and confidence in himself and the therapist are developed. (Abraham, 1974)

Through the therapeutic process the client gradually comes into contact with his inner experience as a separate person and learns to take council with himself. It is this capacity to locate himself and reflect on his inner experience which he internalizes through the dialogue process. It is through the ongoing setting with the therapist, who attends and helps the client to understand, that the client's own capacity to take council with himself is reorganized and strengthened. Through this process he internalizes the capacity to attend to, contain, experience, reflect on and thereby reorganize and transform his own experience. (Freud, 1940)

In terms of movement my focus is to use body work for the purposes of discovering new experience, interpersonal communication and intra-psychic reorganization through insight into meaning, though some reconstitutional work may occur. The actual body work involves many areas of attention: (1) developing the capacity of attending to and identifying aspects of one's experience; (2) locating sensation and movement impulses and any other body feelings; (3) discovering the motions and dynamic movements of tensions as patterns that arise from the inner impulses; (4) such a procedure includes, of course, exploring the range of body functioning and expression as it emerges meaningfully in the therapy, the quality of efforts, tension-relaxation, blocking and the particular function it serves in each specific case, especially in the breathing mechanisms, the expressive meaning of specific gestures, movement qualities and body parts, shape of the body, body image and relationship to gravity, alignment, etc. This also involves developing a language to talk about such non-verbal experiences.

Typically, the client comes in and talks about whatever he chooses. If he so desires, he can start right out with a passage of movement or of body awareness and exploration. Of course it does not happen that way very often, since we are involved with his whole development which includes verbal communication about himself and his life as well. During the conversation I might intervene, picking up on some relevant aspect of his communication which has been expressed subtly in gestures, body tensions, postures or facial expressions. This might be explored and developed for varying lengths of time. A problem might be clarified by focusing on its body aspects in terms of a movement, a series of sensations, as motion-images or in relation to phantasy. Sometimes, asking the client not to do anything but just note what is happening inside his body, provides relevant and useful information. Such listening may mark the beginning of an extended exploration. Frequently, the client will initiate the body work and develop the material according to his own inclinations. The periods of involvement may last a long time or merely consist of momentary reflections which are immediately integrated into the internal flow of experience or into the verbal conversations. There may, or may not, be verbal commenting going on between the client and myself during the body work. I find that sometimes, speaking enhances the process of focusing and associating; other times it disturbs the concentration and flow of experience. The verbal work afterwards may deal with the actual body experience and/or may focus on the associations that emerged. These are only a few examples of how a session might begin and develop. Clearly there is no planned structure beforehand. We just try to articulate what is there, what is obvious but unobserved.

I believe that there is so much going on at every moment which is actual and real in terms of the client's own emotional-mental and body response that I find I do not want to add my own structures and preconceptions. I want to find and work with the events in their authentic form as they emerge spontaneously from the client. The task is to identify accurately what is, in fact, really there "going on." This is, in itself, a very challenging task. This point of view is in keeping with the point of view of dynamically oriented, insight therapist in which it is thought that ongoing attention to what is being presented from moment to moment and session to session will unravel the problems in a way and with a timing that will be therapeutically effective. Some people refer to this as a "process orientation." As the work continues, understanding and experience deepens, the more troubled material emerges, comes to the surface and is faced. This is in contradistinction to methods that delve into the defense system and precipitate emotion by deliberately structured techniques. With flexible interventions that flow with the experience itself, conflicts can be dealt with without any serious threat to the organization of the personality.

Role of the Therapist

It is important to understand that in individual work, in contrast to group work, the intensity of the transference is much greater and more immdiate. In keeping with psychodynamic therapy, I am involved as the therapist with using my capacities for the purpose of assisting the client to experience and know himself as a separate person and in relation to others. I am present for the client to utilize for the purpose of getting to know himself, not for him to use our interaction to get to know who I am. This is in contrast to methods which use the interaction in a direct person-to-person relationship which may include self-revelation, modeling, advice-giving, role-playing, etc. Since I am there for the client to discover himself, I try not to interact directly with the transference reactions and distortions. By reflecting this material back to the client and not interacting with it, I am making his experience the object of our mutual collaboration. The reflective nature of the more limited interaction maintains a focus which doubles back on the client. Thus my work involves trying to sense and communicate what the client is projecting and transfering onto me, or how he might be trying to elicit a desired response from me. I have personally found that these ongoing transference situations can most clearly be defined and separated out as the client's own personal material if I am not making it seem more rooted in external reality by contributing to it, interacting with it or acting it out with him. When I don't enter into his material as he planned, then something new happens. He bumps into himself. Through this therapeutic process the client gradually comes into contact with his inner experience and learns to take council with himself.

For the dance therapist especially there are certain therapeutic dangers in interacting physically with the client. As we all know the physical contribution of movement and body work adds a powerful dimension to the psychotherapy; therefore, which way the movement or body work is used must be evaluated all the more carefully. Manipulation and massage of the body, touch, overt teaching, leading, helping, demonstrating and spontaneously interacting in movement with the client may all be used counter-therapeutically by the client in his attemp to engage the therapist to fulfill unstated and often unconscious longings to be taken care of by the therapist, to be told what to do, or controlled etc., all of which defeat the goals of therapy. The acting out and gratification of longings often keeps these feelings at an unfelt (and unconsciously gratified) level and prevents them from emerging into the therapeutic process. It is so easy, for instance, as therapists, to feel (project) one's own unidentified longings in the client and to try to fulfill them, vicariously attempting to satisfy oneself by trying to satisfy the client. Any promise on the part of the therapist to fulfill these needs is seductive and robs the client of the opportunity to experience the needs and come to terms with them. Touching, holding, leaning, etc., are powerful interactive movement tools, the ramifications of which are much stronger in individual therapy when they occur with the therapist. Certainly some dance therapists do use these methods very effectively even in individual sessions especially to make contact with highly regressed non-verbal patients. What I am suggesting is that care be taken by the dance therapist to determine if these directly "helpful" interactions are being interpreted by the client in his own framework and are being used counter-therapeutically in a fashion other than what is intended.

The following are some examples of the reflective use of movement and verbal observations on my part. While a client Mr. C was verbally recalling and experiencing the very familiar and repetitive situation of being like an outcast in most social situations, he was in touch with the expressions and feelings of embarrassment, wanting to hide and feeling unwanted. But he was not aware that his fist was tensely clenched. When I noted the fact of his fist, that non-verbal aspect came into his consciousness. A rush of anger and feeling of unfairness was felt and then verbally expressed. As this work continued, when more of the situation was included and experienced, he could recognize it for the first time as an acting out of a particular repetitive childhood experience. This spontaneous insight had much emotional impact and meaning for him. The addition of the tense fist into his awareness opened up his experience to aspects of himself with which he was not in contact. There are other times, of course, where such observations might not be so relevant, but then the client usually passes over it and continues with his material.

In addition to verbalizing, at other moments, I might physically reflect or describe what I perceive in the client's body expression. In this sense the client receives my body movements visually and kinesthetically. Schilder (1950) sees this sort of communication as very basic, an essential feature of human exchange. He discusses how body image communicates immediately and directly to body image. In this technique my body is used as well as my words and intonation to identify, locate, reflect back and communicate about aspects of the client's communication. It must be remembered however, that for some clients such reflective methods are not appropriate if, for instance, they are taken as invasive, controlling, too intense or overwhelming.

Working with non-verbal experiences does not mean just working with movement. During the sessions, I may spend part of the time just watching the client in his own process of exploring. For some clients this presents many difficulties and requires working through important material having to do with my watching. Also, the client's experience of my presence and whatever that may mean to him is an ever present issue that is frequently dealt with. I cannot emphasize enough that much of the therapeutic work occurs by working with the subtle transference reactions and projections that are indirectly communicated verbally and non-verbally.

Case Study

I have selected various sessions with Mr. C. to illustrate some of the theoretical material which has been discussed throughout this chapter. This example is not intended to serve as a complete case study nor does it represent the client's whole psychodynamic constellation of therapeutic development.

Mr. C. is working successfully as a professional. He is in his early forties. He had already been in about two years of group and individual psychotherapy when he first started working with me and has continued with this throughout the period that we had been working together. I saw him once a week for a fifty minute session. He was single at the time. His two marriages were without children and ended in divorce.

When I first started working with Mr. C., he was continually experiencing his social life as uncomfortable and embarrasing. He often found himself unable to have anything to say. To him it seemed as if there were "no thoughts." He felt inadequate and was afraid he would be laughed at. He was always looking to see what others did and was trying to imitate them as if they knew something that he did not know. He had these feelings with me and expected me to structure his movements for him, as if he did not know how. He was always trying to figure out what to do or say as if he could find some key or answer that would enable him to know what to do, and how to be spontaneous. If a woman he was dating would talk to someone else at a gathering and not to him, he would feel even more unbearably uncomfortable and would have to leave. Many of these repetitious experiences did not have any meaning to him.

Though he superficially knew some facts about his first six years, he remembered very little. Until he was six, he and his brother were brought up in the home nursery with the two very Catholic nurse maids. The children rarely left the nursery. He could recall how even the thought of being outside the walls was scary. According to him they rarely saw their parents except for special occasions, quick hello's and goodbye's and occasionally when being shown off by their parents to other adults. The pervasiveness of his repression and depression severely reduced his capacity to experience himself and his life. He felt impoverished and was, in fact, impoverished in thought, image, feeling and a sense of intention, purpose and meaning. He had little memory of his past, did not remember his dreams except occasionally when he might recall a seemingly meaningless fragment.

At the time of the following session, I had seen Mr. C. a number of months. Since what he felt to be a more successful vacation, he had begun to become more aware of the difference between his usual experience of himself and how he felt on the vacation. During the vacation he felt he had attained a more relaxed, peaceful yet alive state of inactivity which was quite different from his usual "inert," "dead-like" feeling. He felt that he would usually strive for the inert feeling whenever given the opportunity. In the course of verbal discussion and recollection, the actual inert quality became more immediate and available to consciousness at that moment as direct physical experience. His dread was of sinking into this inert state which, according to his self-concept, was an expression of his real self. He was sure that spontaneous action was not natural to him and that he had to push himself to get going; though he knew that once he had pushed himself, he would enjoy it. As he spoke, I began to mention out loud what his body was doing, asking him to pay attention to it and see what he could discover. What was quite apparent was the continual and alternating efforts of tightening and pulling in his shoulder, across the chest, arms, and then the whole torso. The impression I had was that these fairly small but actually quite effortful tensions were inhibiting not only any possibility of a more relaxed or easy state, but that they were constraining and covering any spontaneous motions toward action. They contributed to his body image and self concept of "inertness." This is a clear example of how tension can be utilized to change the nature of one's experience, self-perception and self-image.

As he focused on what was happening, this became very evident to him. He could easily feel the many efforts he was making to hold himself in. When he realized this, he then became interested in finding out what would happen when he let go of these various holdings; he wanted to find out what was being held back. This led to a passage of exploration which consisted of following the sensations in his body as they represented themselves, first with following his awareness and locating the different muscular places which he was holding, letting them go and then noting the small twinges of sensation that occurred. Once he began to let go of the constrictions, the sensations that he felt were impulses toward as yet undefined motions in different muscles.

As Mr. C. attended to these undifferentiated twinges throughout his body, they became more and more defined, gradually becoming actual impulses to twitch and to make very small stretches. The sensation was itchy as if these small movements were like scratching the itch. The whole experience was quite new to him. This pulling, stretching, squirming continued for two or three more sessions. As it developed, the movements became fuller, larger and more forceful, but still very much in the restrained "pulling" mode. It felt good to him to feel the resistance against the floor, to push and strain. He also began to feel with more clarity how much counter-effort he used to resist the impulses toward spontaneous motion. Though this seemed to strain him, the effortful pushing and pulling gave him a feeling of aliveness and strength. He became aware that there was a definite inhibition of free unbounded impulses or motion.

A session or so later, Mr. C. announced how frustrated he felt. Now he did not like the feeling of staying put, of inactivity, but he did not know what he wanted to do. This is a psychological statement which correlates with the physical expression in the last session, in which he had moved from a feeling of inertness toward an impulse for action and resultant frustration. The physical impulses were also felt to be undefined and therefore difficult to satisfy.

In this example, Mr. C. had already attained a capacity for work at a more advanced level in terms of using the body work therapeutically. He was able to sense and develop his experiences with a good deal of articulation. That is, he was able to locate by feel his sensations and impulses, and he was able to identify and follow them. It was much more difficult for him to do this with his mental associations. Initially, just finding anything mental to say was very difficult. Therapeutically, even the very process of having to articulate about his immediate experience was developing in him the capacity to find a language for his inner experiences and helping him to link his subjective experiencing self to his objective observing self. This also helped to develop his capacity to take council with himself and to communicate his inner self to the outside world.

As can be seen in this example, all four aspects may occur almost simultaneously, alternately, or separately within one session or over an extended period of time. In the example cited above, his "experiencing self" initially felt; then his "observing self" identified the inertness that had been subjectively "happening" to him. Until this time, he had accepted this as his "natural state." It formed the basis of his body image and self concept. Initially, he was not in contact with any of the mechanisms by which his action self was holding back and inhibiting any spontaneous impulses. Once Mr. C. was able to identify his action, in constricting his impulses, he could begin to experiment with changing it. Though he was still at the beginning of this passage of work, the integrating self was already linking up the experiencing, observing and the action aspects of his experience thus enabling a new organization to emerge.

A few sessions later, Mr. C. came five minutes late. He wanted to understand this new tendency toward lateness since recently it had been occuring in everything that he was doing. He was rather perplexed since for the last number of years he had made a big effort and had been effective in taking active charge of his time. He had always felt very good about this punctuality. During the discussion he began to identify that it did not seem to be related to a feeling about where he was going, nor about who or what he was meeting. It felt non-specific. All he could identify was a feeling of ignoring time and slowing down whenever he was about to go anywhere.

At this point, I suggested he try some body work and suggested he set up in his imagination some places in the room to go to, paying attention to the feelings and inclinations inside himself regarding "leaving" and "going." I noted that perhpas there wouldn't be any actual movement but just imaginings or small impulses, "toward" or "away" or "whatever." He spent a long time just sitting and feeling. Then he moved slowly from place to place stopping and starting. Occasionally he would comment on his experience. It became quite clear to him that he "did not want to leave" from wherever he was. It didn't matter where he was; he felt much more comfortable and secure staying. Being in a place was always better than going. He liked best the huge, nine-foot wooden, carved chest at the far end of the room.* In between these two, he felt very exposed. Whenever he would arrive at either the table or the chest, he would lean on them. He felt safer there. He especially liked the "enveloping" feeling at the chest. He explored the carved wood with a great sensitivity and tenderness. When leaning against it his whole body would become less caved in. He squatted at the base of it, making himself very small, feeling its big enveloping quality. When he would leave the chest, his body would become harder; his own chest would go back into its characteristic sunken carriage with his hands in his pocket and his shoulders raised. To me it looked as if he were using his back to provide a cloak for himself under which he could huddle. When he was being protected by the chest, he would no longer appear huddled; his chest would lift, and even though he was leaning on it there was actually much less restraint throughout his entire torso. This exploration lasted for a long time with many slow and faltering passages back and forth across the room and back to the chest.

*The sessions were held in my medium sized living-room with plants in the corner, moveable pillows and no furniture except the large chest at one end of the room with a small dining area at the other end of the living room.

He felt there was "something towering and protective" about it. But he would also move away from it when he felt "over-pretected and restrained." As he wandered around, he realized that he would go back to the chest as "home base." He reminded himself of a "child in a new situation who would wander away from it and back again." The chest as "mother" was obvious to him, though very surprising since he had no memories of such a mother and was, in fact, brought up in a wealthy European home in which he had nothing but occasional contact with his "busy white-gloved mother" and Catholic nursemaids until he was six. He has few memories of his nursery days of maids except that the best thing he could do was "not to cause any trouble." He was able to remember how he always felt that "God was watching all the time." He felt he would go to hell forever if he did anything wrong. Though perplexed about this protective experience with the chest, he could not deny it. He could vividly feel that something inside himself knew what this experience was and had reconstructed it, though he could not contact any direct memory of it. He noted what a kindly and reassuring protective feeling the chest gave him and that he had been feeling more insecure recently. He made the link with the house and his secure business, both of which had that protective feeling. He had been planning for these last few years of arranging his finances so that he would be free from his professional work. But as he was beginning to move out of that inertness and to feel the impulses away from the secure professional position he had established, he felt scared. At one time, he had "felt good about doing nothing," now he wants to get going but he doesn't know what he wants.

This material suggests a development from the last sessions where he worked with a feeling of holding back through tension in his body. Now, he is aware of holding back in time, space and in his life. Without going into the psychodynamics of this session, I hope it is clear to the reader that the body experience serves as an opportunity for free association thereby bringing into play some of his internal life, his internal objects and relation to them as well as to his external circumstances. It is by following the material and associations Mr. C. presented and not introducing a prescribed activity, that he arrived where he did.

In the following session, Mr. C. and I talked the entire time about the material that emerged from this last session. It turned out to be his first conscious experience of the dependent longings which, though they had been observed by others, he had never experienced. He still wondered at how he could form such an attachment to the chest since he had no memories of ever forming such an attachment with his real mother. He remembered the many sessions with me previously in which he had explored what he had come to recognize as a constant feeling that he is "encased and shielded." In this session, Mr. C. began to link much of the material we had been exploring over a number of months. His tendency to see others as "knowing" and himself as not knowing and to follow them, his tendency to want them to tell him what to do, and then to feel resentful and controlled by them. At that time, he was already well aware of his anger at feeling controlled, but he had not felt his desire to be controlled. He enumerated many examples with his present girl friend of over-reacting angrily to her wishes to "do" for him. He saw "how any feeling of dependency feels like being controlled." He saw what a bind he put himself in since he felt that "asking for anything brings up the issue of who's in charge and invites someone to control" him. We began to explore how these feelings manifest in the sessions with me. He could now recognize what has become a familiar feeling of wanting to be told what to do, his desire for me and others to give answers, to structure him, to take care of him. He recognized the feeling of not being capable of making his own decisions, as if he is missing something. I suggested that he attributed to me, what feels like the missing and needed knowledge or direction which he felt would enable him to know what he wanted to do and how to do it. Mr. C. identified the feeling of constantly losing himself in his numerous short relationships with women. He realized how he was constantly "switching programs" to suit whichever woman he was going with. He could change his habits according to them, subject himself to their control and resent it deeply. For Mr. C., allowing himself to feel his yearnings was experienced as a temptation which would then threaten to entrap him. Numerous sessions since have been devoted to this desire for and fear of being protectively enveloped, lovingly cuddled an literally entrapped. He could see how he felt safe to invest the chest and other objects, not people, with the yearned for qualities so as to protect himself from surrendering control to them.

Mr. C's tendency to act out his internal object-relations with inanimate objects rather than persons became more evident in the following session in which he discussed his intense reaction when the painter in his apartment removed all of his collected objects. He tearfully realized that all the many objects which clutter up his rooms represent the relationships, and events of his life with which he had lost touch. In short, they represented his relationships, his history and reminded him that he existed. He couldn't stand the thought of discarding his objects. He was surprised to discover how much of his contact with his own experiences transpired unbeknownst to himself through the objects. He had previously felt himself to be devoid of these feelings. Mr. C. reported how he had consciously tried to get rid of any temptation to be possessive, to feel a sense of continuity, of belonging, of cherishing his interpersonal experiences. He felt he had consciously worked very hard on "trying to accept that nothing lasts, especially relationships," trying to live every day in the present like a new day "as if there was no past." Inside himself, he was recreating the emptiness, emotional deprivation, loss and struggles in his childhood and in his present-day, internal life. In this process, affect, thought and meaning were all beginning to emerge and to be linked together, reorganized in a meaningful way.

Three sessions later, Mr. C. brought up his angry reactions to drivers who "can just do what they want." He was very conscious of the resentful feeling that "he can't do what he wants." He felt that he would like to continue with the body work, by just starting and finding out if he can let himself do what he wants, seeing what he wants to do; and if his worst fantasy occurred, that is, that nothing would happen, then he would lie on the floor and just wait until something happened even if he had to endure fifteen minutes. And so with a good deal of patient determintion he began.

He eased slowly down onto the floor allowing and feeling the small adjustments of his body. After awhile everything quieted down except a few very subtle motions in his fingers. Even they stopped moving. And he waited. From my view he seemed to be very focused and attentive. His breathing patterns adjusted, he seemed to be sensing a good deal. Gradually, a very slight and gentle stirring began to occur in his fingers, an easy motion without stretching and without engaging in his usual simultaneous resistance from the antagonist muscles. But then, as is typical with him, he began to stretch and pull with larger more external muscles in isometric movement. He continued in this way throughout his entire body including his breathing patterns. Then, he eased back onto the floor with a gentle unstrained flow in his movement quality. And again, back into the stretching and pulling, but this time with more intensity and pushing and straining. The pushing and straining led to pushing as hard as he could against the wall. He decided to use the hallway so as to be able to exert all of his force from both directions. At some point during this,

I asked him to be alert to any images, thoughts or fantasies. On a number of occasions, he would become especially cautious when the walls creaked. He also tried kicking the wall with a pillow in between, but again seemed to stop the action before completion.

After awhile, right after exerting a hugh amount of force against the walls in the hallway, he reported a fantasy of being in a box and trying to push open the walls. At that point, he had for the first time a "momentary flash of an image of a very authoritarian male face," which he didn't recognize. He couldn't tell whether it was disapproving or stern, whether he was pushing against it or whether it was a spectator to what he was doing. When we later talked about his experience, I noted the times he hesitated and wondered if he was afraid of breaking my house or damaging my pillows. He replied that he was afraid that he would "kick the pillow to bits and tear it apart and that he would crack the plaster." He began to realize how he would have liked "to tear the whole thing down," but at the same time, if he "moves outside the box or plastic bag" he "wouldn't know what to do," that the box is a "prison and shield at the same time." He exclaimed how for "an instant" he felt "a tremendous amount of force which might escalate and escalate." He didn't know which was the most fearful, "getting beat up or hurting others."

Mr. C. felt very pleased with himself for having such an experience. He claimed to have never experienced such a feeling, that he had "never been physical before." The few times he had forced himself to go to the gym he had to force himself into exertion that felt dreary and unpleasant. This material demonstrates how Mr. C's internal life has been externalized and even acted out spatially. The feeling of being encased is a strong and constant one for him, as well as the fear and desire to break through it. This is an integral part of his body image as well.

He returned to the previous subject commenting that "the world beyond the nursery walls seemed so scary and tempting, and now the world outside the (his own) barriers is so scary." He "wants to try to push down the barriers." He couldn't "tell whether the face was disapproving or not." I suggested that the face was a symbol of the God he was always fearfully worrying about in his nursery room days, the God who was always felt to be watching and ready to punish. I wondered at how confused he must have felt then not knowing whether God, or perhaps the nursemaid, would approve or disapprove. That was a familiar feeling to him. It seemed that he didn't understand the rules. He replied that his "one real recollection was of confusion." Then he would "spend hours not knowing what was right or what was wrong, always trying to decide in his mind what to do before taking action." He claimed that he "never played" or acted spontaneously. This lack of spontaneity, holding in and stopping himself both in his thoughts and actions is, of course, the same behavior with which we had been working.

Even in the session just discussed, Mr. C. was still quite removed from the aggressive and destructive impulses which were being expressed there. Not until many months later were his yearnings, fears and destructive feelings felt in the emotional context of his relationships. Many sessions were spent on his emotional removal from me, and on his fear of me expressed in his body as a tendency to "duck and weave" to get away from anticipated blows he expected from me even though he "rationally" knew better. His capacity now to have meaningful and satisfying experiences within himself and in relation to others, has been greatly enriched, especially in his primary relation to the woman about whom he is serious. He began to feel and directly express his needs for intimacy and tenderness with much less concern about being controlled and entrapped. He began to be able to feel the extremity of his rage when he re-enacted his childhood feelings and fantasies of being neglected. In the process, he also started remembering his dreams which have become well developed, complex and emotionally expressive. After a few months his next steps involved a new sense of mastery and excitement in exploring and achieving a fuller physical functioning and pleasure, range of body action and improved alignment.

In this work evolving from the focus on alignment, Mr. C. was able to identify what to him felt like the source of his own ugliness and unacceptableness—the feeling of a great nauseating evil inside himself, his own violent and sadistic fantasies of hurting and damaging others. We discussed the anxiety he felt at being exposed to me in the alignment work and how criticized he felt internally when he looked at something wrong with himself. This feeling that something is wrong with his body turned out to be an ever-present fear. At this point in the conversation his body began to go into the familiar drawn in, hunched over posture. When I called his attention to it, he let the impulse develop. He began to feel nauseated and identified the feeling and posture as the evil, gnarled malicious sense of himself that he was always trying to hide and contain. He felt this to be at his "core." Even then it was too painful an awareness. He felt fearfully unable to share the actual destructive fantasies he was in contact with in his own thoughts. But he was able to see how he makes himself impotent in the face of any confrontation, confusing any aggression within himself as this very threatening evil self. He reported having had such a feeling surge through his body when in an argument with his woman the night before. His rage wasn't just that he wanted to hit her; he wanted to completely destroy her, obliterate her when he felt that she was treating him "as if she didn't give a damn" about him, like in the old days with his family. He made himself impotent in the face of this rage. No wonder Mr. C. has complained of not being spontaneous and of being out of touch with any natural aggression or assertive direction. His body with which he felt something was "wrong" expressed and contained the "bad" and dangerous impulses which he felt make him so unacceptable.

In this session, Mr. C. showed much more integration. He was able to tolerate contact with what is for him very threatening internal fantasies and to link them up to feelings and behaviors in relation to both his present and past significant relations. He was also able to discriminate between the woman of his present relationship onto whom he is projecting his internal fantasies and the fantasied female object as it is located within himself. For the first time since I had known him, he was showing the capacity for healthy guilt as concern for another. He stated how he had never understood in group when a particular man felt badly because of his aggression and his fear of hurting someone. Mr. C. had always thought the man was deceiving himself and that he was really just afraid for himself out of fear of retaliation or rejection (persecutory guilt). This time Mr. C. understood what it is to be really concerned about hurting the other person. He felt a sense of shame about his own destructiveness and began to understand what it was about himself that felt so ugly and unacceptable. The deeper contact with this fearful aspect of himself brought him a good deal of relief and enabled him to funtion on a new level.

This case illustrates some of the values of focusing on the body and following the cues and impulses so minutely. So much of Mr. C's experience was threatening, repressed from consciousness and partially expressed through the body in unconscious behavior and incipient action without being linked to awareness, to self perception or thought. In such a case as Mr. C., when the body information is so divergent from his self concept, the body experience assists in the process of reclaiming some of what had been repressed. As the material was becoming more articulated and linked coherently to image, thought, memory and emotion, it began to have more meaning. This series of sessions demonstrates the overlapping and ongoing development of material in the process of internal change. As the material emerges it is subjectively experienced, identified and made an object of reflection, thereby enabling it to be linked up to related associations to be integrated into the present ongoing structure. Each new linkage and integration brings about a slightly new constellation from which the next experience emerges.

Bibliography

Abraham, J., Psycho-Analyst, 1974, Personal Communications, San Diego, California.

Bion, W.R. "Differentiation of the Psychotic from the Non-Psychotic Personalities." In Bion, W.R., *Second Thoughts,* London: Heinemann, 1957.

Fletcher, D. "The Use of Movement and Body Experience in Therapy." In *Therapeutic Process: Movement As Integration,* Proceedings of Ninth Annual Conference, American Dance Therapy Association, Columbia: Maryland, 1974.

Freud, S. *The Ego and the Id.* London: Hogarth Press, Ltd, 1927.

———. *New Introductory Lectures on Psychoanalysis.* (1933), New York: W.W. Norton & Co. Inc., 1965.

———. *An Outline of Psychoanalysis* (1940). New York: W.W. Norton & Co. Inc., 1949.

Guntrip, H. *Personality Structure and Human Interaction.* New York: International Universities Press, Inc., 1961.

Hunt, V.V. "Neuromuscular Organization in Emotional States." In *What Is Dance Therapy, Really*? Proceedings of the Seventh Annual Conference, American Dance Therapy Association, Columbia: Maryland, 1972.

Isaacs, S. "The Nature and Function of Phantasy." (1943) In Jones E., ed. *Developments in Psycho-Analysis,* London: The Hogarth Press, 1952.

———. *Social Development in Young Children.* (1933) New York: Schocken Books, 1972.

Jacobson, E. *Biology of Emotions.* Springfield, Illinois: Charles Thomas Publisher, 1967.

Klein, M. *The Psycho-Analysis of Children.* (1933) Delacorte Press/Seymour Lawrence, 1975.

———. *Love, Guilt and Reparation & Other Works 1921–1945.* Delacorte Press/Seymour Lawrence, 1975.

———. *Envy and Gratitude & Other Works 1946–1963.* Delacorte Press/Seymour Lawrence, 1975.

Rado, S. *Adaptational Psychodynamics: Motivation and Control.* New York: Science House, 1969.

Reich, W. *Character Analysis.* (1933) New York: Simon and Schuster, 1972.

Rolf, I.P. "Structural Integration: Postural Release." In *The Journal of the Institute for the Comparative Study of History, Philosophy and the Sciences,* Coombe Springs, England: Vol. I, No. I, June Issue, 1963.

Rush, S.B. Psychologist, Personal Communications, Los Angeles, California, 1974.

Saul, L.J. *Psychodynamically Based Psychotherapy.* New York: Science House, 1972.

Schilder, P. *The Image and Appearance of the Human Body.* New York: John Wiley and Sons, Inc., 1950.

Chapter 10

MOVEMENT THERAPY: A TRANSPERSONAL-TRANSFORMATIONAL APPROACH

*Barbara Freudenthal Govine, MA, DTR**

Genesis

In the beginning I loved to move. My favorite childhood memories are of active, spontaneous play. My total self found great joy in running like the wind down the hill to Lake Michigan. I recall the exhuberance of challenging gravity by swinging on vines in the ravines. I knew, from my deepest place of knowing, that my birthright included living in a body which could experience and express my deepest thoughts and feelings. It was through my body that I understood my relationship to nature. It was through my body that I understood my relationship to God.

In my teens I learned that vitality and endurance were basic to my core nature. My love of movement took the form of exhilarating expression through tennis, cycling and long-distance hiking. College was my time to dance. I had to love affair with modern dance.

UCLA in the early 50's meant delighting in the inspriational teaching of Valerie Hunt who helped me establish by science base. She opened doors to my beginning explorations of body image. A beacon light shone for me in Marian Chace's early articles and I knew that I too would be using movement as a bridge between worlds and realities. I was also drawn to studies in psychology and group process.

I married for the first time while still an undergraduate and when my children were very young I began working in movement with nursery school children, being particularly drawn to the creativity of their free spirits. Later my increasing interest in multi levels of communication led me to work in movement with emotionally disturbed adults.

Simultaneously it was my great fortune to have the opportunity for study and continued relationships with three of the pioneers of dance therapy—Trudi Schoop, Mary Whitehouse and Marian Chace. I was profoundly influenced by each of these charismatic teachers.

From Trudi I learned a deep appreciation of the use of humor in a therapeutic exchange and the value of using the group as a support system. From Mary I learned the potency of giving voice to dream material and the powerful impact of working one-to-one in therapy. From Marian I learned enormous respect for the importance of timing in making interventions and developing discernment in knowing what movements, feelings and statements to "pick up" and develop.

*Barbara Freudenthal Govine, MA, DTR, is a transpersonal movement therapist in private practice, a licensed family counselor and a certified practitioner of essential integration, an evolutionary body work approach.

Theoretical Model

These are my basic assumptions for a transpersonal-transformational model. I believe human beings are here for a purpose, that they are a part of a universal plan. I believe each individual is in the process of becoming who he or she really is. Each travels this journey in a unique way that reflects the nature of the essential self. Each is reaching for completion of the essential evolution relative to this plane.

In this process of transcendence each in one's own, personal metaphor embraces the divinity within. Each discovers the relationship to his/her higher self. The journey of self, soul or essence is one of ultimate merging with the higher self. I refer to that part of the self that knows the individual's perfection and relationship to the universe. The higher self operates as a compassionate observer, holding a template of each person's ultimate refinement. The higher self is an inner source of wisdom and purpose.

Magnetism is the organizing principle on this plane. It is through magnetism that one attracts to oneself what is needed for completion of each progressing step in one's process (Winer, 1975-8). The entire drama is played out in a climate of free will. The full capacity to choose experiences that foster growth, self knowledge and enlightenment is present within each person. The total self—mind, body and spirit—have vast information regarding what is needed for higher consciousness.

What is superbly valuable is to have access to a mode for integrating personal metaphors, images and experience. Transpersonal-transformational movement therapy is one such mode.

I believe the individual develops in an organized, sequential fashion, mastering the various thought forms that are encountered in each life processes. All thought forms are some aspect of love. Integrity, loyalty and courage are examples of the many thought forms that must be fully comprehended before the journey to self-realization can be completed.

A transpersonal-transformational approach is compatible with a developmental approach, and what makes movement therapy such a potent force is the continual opportunity it provides to tap into this fund of developmental information.

We carry with us knowledge of earlier phases of development.

> "Long before man reaches the verbal stage he goes through what we will call the 'occupational' stage which is formed by touch, sense communication and movement. In this 'occupational phase' man is taking control over the various functions of his body. His soul enters his body, so to speak, and provides it with its functions which will forever serve as a resonance chamber for all his feelings" (Derbolowsky, 1964, p. 5).

Memory traces of earlier experiences and relationships are retained. These memories are stored in the body on the cellular level. The fascia, the connective tissue which holds the body together and envelops all the muscle and internal organs, is a primary medium for retaining this information (Rolf, 1973). Fascia carries multilevel messages and gives structure to essence (Locks, 1977-78).

Memory traces are not limited to muscles and sensory organs but extend to every nerve cell and every organic element of the body. Imprints of experience in the preverbal stage can influence visual experience, bodily sensation and total behavior (Lewis, 1974).

Imprints of information, especially parental messages, injunctions and attributions, concerning oneself and one's body are cellularly retained as well. How one moves reflects a composite of one's history—one's experiences as a part of a family, a culture, a universe. One's body reflects how an individual was touched as an infant, was regarded in one's family, and was taught about the body and self worth. One's body reflects the people one has loved, the joys one has embraced, the losses one has sustained—the cumulative effect of each individual's life journey.

Individuals manifest themselves in their bodies; the body is the visual representation of the total being. The body reflects the splits and the unities of the total self.

Movement is behavior that reflects personal and total functioning of body, mind and spirit. Movement is energy being manifested. Through movement a range covering the spectrum of fluid, essential expression to blocked, split, linear expression can be exhibited.

Health

Health is more than having a body that works well. It is feeling good about oneself, dealing creatively with the people and situations in one's life, and growing spiritually towards a sense of wholeness. Thus from a transpersonal-transformational perspective health encompasses self, society and cosmos.

Health reflects itself in dynamic balance of energy. By energy I mean the vital life force which animates all things. I am talking about what is identified as "ki" or "chi" or "prana" in various Eastern philosophies and systems of energy awareness.

In optimum health, all of the body's energy centers and pathways are available for response to the moment. In the body's state of vibrant health, fascia is resilient, neither restricting the flow of movement nor being so open as to be lacking definition.

One of the key roles of a movement therapist is to assist a person in finding a balance of his or her energy flow. A person's breathing pattern, movement style and symbolic movement are some of the observable factors. The movement therapist also refines intuitive information and learns to process subtle sensory cues in comprehending a person's energy state.

Full functioning as revealed in the body means having access to a variety of options and possibilities. Full humanness includes the ability to find pleasure in movement and in one's freely functioning body.

Each body possesses cellular knowledge of this state of fluid energy. Each cell contains holographic information of the bodies' perfection. However, sometimes the cells act as though they are experiencing a lapse of memory of their hologram. Dance therapy offers one path for remembering this perfect blueprint.

Trudi Schoop writes eloquently on this subject.

> "I envision a being, still in Paradise, living in joyous confirmation of itself, in accordance with its birth, its life and its death, and proud of its ability to perpetuate its own image. It is a human form as it was meant to be and to function, in its complete, perfect state—revelling in its breathing, exulting in its motion, beautifully assertive in its total involvement with existence." (p. 39)

Dysfunction

Dysfunction is experienced as being cut off from one's sense of self. Frequently people report an awareness that something is missing, that they know something more is available to them but they can't connect with it.

In this place of dis-ease people rarely communicate with self, let alone the energy of higher self and the rhythm of the universe. They appear to be out of touch with their sense of purpose and their path for expression of their unique nature.

I am reminded of a woman in therapy who had the repeated experience that she learned by doing things backwards; and in many of her movement sequences, she literally backed into spaces. She felt this pattern kept getting in her way of finding her course or direction. Much of our work together was spent in discovering her picture of unity in which she experienced forward, progressive movement in her process.

Often in dysfunction a body area is restricted, denied or overemphasized. Frequently the location of the area is indicative of the messages a person carries from earlier experience. It is no accident that one person sustains great tension in the neck and shoulders, another restricts mobility on the whole left side and another experiences tightening in the abdominal area.

Dance therapy involves decoding someone else's language, much of which is spoken without words. It involves making sense out of body language and all the nuances of non-verbal communication. Dance therapy often involves finding the missing pieces of a personal jigsaw which have remained hidden or obscure in other life and therapeutic encounters.

Therapy

Therapy is a continuous evolutionary process reaching towards a person's highest creative potential. It begins where a person is and moves towards alignment with their essential nature. A transpersonal-transformational approach to movement therapy uses body awareness and movement to facilitate the knowing of this evolving sense of unity.

This facilitation continually takes place in the vibration or quality of the next step of a person's process. Transpersonal-transformational movement therapy works at the level of the resolution rather than at the level of the problem.

I used to work on the problem level. For example, if a client brought to a session her rage towards her mother, I would have been likely to create a safe space for her to find cathartic expression. My intent would have been to facilitate insight and change, working with the polarities involved. Today if I were presented with the same situation I would first bring myself to total presence with the person. In that moment I often receive a sense of the next step the person is to work on. In this example of rage the next step might be compassion. If so it would be the configuration of compassion I would orchestrate rather than anger, aiming toward an evolving synthesis and harmony.

Role of the Therapist

Treatment is made possible by providing a safe relationship with a conscious, caring therapist. Since the problems and distortions a person brings to therapy usually represent an expression of his view of himself, his body and his world, treatment involves an examination of these beliefs within a relationship with an intuitive, aware person.

Successful treatment requires the therapist to have access to the kind of caring known as "high indifference" (Joy, 1976). In the state of high indifference the therapist is able to view the problem from above the level of the conflict without projection or identification. The therapist holds in his or her own thought the vibration or quality of the resolution.

Treatment in this dimension permits the therapist to bring caring and empathy to their highest form. High indifference combines the gifts of compassion and objectivity. When I touch this state of consciousness I feel the most aligned with my own higher self. And I feel wonder and gratitude for the experience.

For treatment to be successful the therapist must be totally present. The therapist must be fully there—in the moment—with the client.

Ronald Laing (1967) shines further light on this sense of presence in the therapeutic relationship.

> "Psychotherapy is an activity in which that aspect of the patient's being, his relatedness to others, is used for therapeutic ends. The therapist acts on the principle that, since relatedness is potentially present in everyone, that he may not be wasting his time in sitting for hours with a silent catatonic who gives every evidence that he does not recognize his existence" (p. 26).

In providing this therapeutic connection, the therapist is forever mindful that the client has selected his behavior for his own purposes, be they conscious or unconscious. Therefore the client will modify, change or let go of this pattern—or leap to a new space—only when and if he is ready. The client may believe, either consciously or unconsciously, that the work he needs to do to resolve the problem may be more difficult than the pain of the problem itself. The client always needs to be aware of his choice and free will.

I reflect on my immense learning from being a therapist in a cancer research project. The primary goal of the project was to facilitate transformation. Several of the patients reached the point of clarity where they determined that the effort they needed to put into "cleaning up" relationships and reducing stress was greater than they chose to expand. They then made conscious choices to embrace the cancer rather than attempt to alter its course.

Treatment, at its core, involves examining one's belief system. Therapy encourages the client to make connections with messages which have been internalized and restrictions which have been embodied. It is not enough to merely experience the blocking, splitting and holding back. For these patterns to be dealt with in a process leading to change they must be seen in relation to one's life style and one's system of beliefs.

It is not easy to openly look at one's basic beliefs and values. This is often unknown or frightening territory. It is much easier to protect oneself with the ideal image that one has of oneself.

Maslow (1971) expresses his concern for

> "those portions of ourselves which are rejected and relegated to unconscious existence but can and eventually do break through . . . affecting our perceptions as well as our actions" (p. 157).
>
> "We protect ourselves and our ideal image of ourselves by repression and similar defenses, which are essentially techniques by which we avoid becoming conscious of unpleasant or dangerous truths" (p. 60).

Treatment Process

Treatment involves using fantasy, dream and meditation material to tap into the creative process. A transpersonal-transformational approach encourages dialogues with one's higher self, first to contact and then incorporate clear knowledge of one's essential nature.

Movement provides an open channel for retrieving unconscious, unedited material. Bringing the content which emerges from fantasy work into the therapeutic situation permits one to see the world fresh rather than with prejudged perceptions. Employing fantasy explorations is like looking with Zen eyes to see for the first time, much in the way a young child makes initial discovery.

Movement therapy offers an extraordinary opportunity to combine the story and the symbolism of dream and meditation material with a form that can be examined, explored and developed. Movement therapy is a framework for making messages tangible and meaningful as they emerge from the unconscious. My work has expanded this paradigm to include transformational messages from both the higher and lower unconscious (Russell, 1977).

Dreams are "befriended" (Hillman, 1967). The dreamer is afforded a nurturing climate to put into movement the various voices of the dreams or meditations. Movement therapy also introduces a unique setting in which to create a new ending to one's dreams.

The client may elect to use movement therapy as an avenue for conversing with his or her higher self. Clients report profound insights after an experience of moving in this transpersonal energy. I recall one young woman who identified the energy of her higher self as maternal, nurturing and symbolic of the highest attainment. Repeatedly her image was of a large, robed figure beckoning her to come closer, to get to know her better.

Transpersonal movement therapy encourages the expression of humor and the experience of play as a part of the healing process. There is no law of the universe that says that one must suffer in order to grow. Therapy need not be all serious and somber! To quote Golas, (1971):

> "It's all right to have a good time. That is one of the most important messages of enlightenment. We should try to comprehend the highest pleasure level, the pleasure of God, so to speak, in all that we perceive. No one in higher consciousness wants any of us to have a miserable time on earth" (P. 30).

Transpersonal-transformational therapy is concerned with finding a balance in one's energy flow and one's life. This can be seen as establishing a balance in all of the body's energy centers and pathways. Often one or more of these areas is blocked or barely functioning. Movement therapy provides experiences for bringing the body and therefore the total person into fine tuning, such as one would tune an exquisite musical instrument.

Some clients are in need of a sense of grounding. They literally have lost their connection with the earth. Movement therapy offers one way to reestablish this basic survival relationship.

Other clients may be blocked in a sense of owning their own power. Movement therapy becomes a treatment of choice for working through and claiming these energies, always in the context of the bigger picture. Even though I am aware of blocking of parts I consistently work for at least a glimpse of the overview.

In the transpersonal-transformational approach to movement therapy I function as a model who respects and values my body as a person who finds pleasure, meaning and intimacy in relationships. It is through my living example of the esteem in which I place my own fluid body that those who consult with me are reminded of the freedom and pleasure they too once knew, no matter how briefly. It is through the value I place on personal relationships and my relationship to God that I serve as a guide to a greater sense of meaning to life.

I am a participant/observer who shares what I see in a thoughtful, caring way. My aim is to function compassionately and objectively. I believe the therapist must function in the therapeutic relationship as a real, authentic person worthy of an investment of trust on the part of the client. The therapist clearly needs to have done and continue to do a great deal of personal work. As Ram Dass reminds us, "Therapy is only as high as the therapist" (1974, p. 20).

Case Study

The following case study summarizes individual movement therapy with a 19 year-old man over a four-month period of time. My work was done in a transpersonal-transformational mode. The client was hospitalized voluntarily in a psychiatric unit within a private, acute hospital. He had no history of previous hospitalization.

Sessions were scheduled once a week for 45-minute time periods. In addition to dance therapy the client was involved in individual and group psychotherapy, art therapy, sociodrama and the overall ward mileu.

Ken was admitted to the unit after he attempted to overdose of a large amount of medication which he had available at home. He described the period immediately prior to taking the pills as one in which he was preoccupied with concerns of good and evil. He called this his "God thing" and he was terrified with the thought that he would project evil onto and into other people.

On first contant Ken presented a "frozen" facial expression which had feeling qualities of extreme withdrawal, immobility, fear and panic. Occasionally he would display an inappropriate smile.

Ken made limited use of space. For a young man of tall, athletic build he moved in a hesitant, tentative manner with only hints of reaching out to explore his environment. Eye contact was difficult for him to establish and maintaim. He spoke in a flat monotone and rarely verbalized more than three or four words in sequence.

Our initial connection was established through discovering the music and sounds to which he liked to listen. Ken clarified that he turned most music into "background" noise but we found that he was responsive to recordings of environmental sounds (ocean waves, animal sounds, wind and rain sounds).

Sessions began to develop a pattern. Most often they would start with an active, athletic-like warm-up in which Ken would teach me "exercises" he had learned in high school. This appeared to make contact with the healthy part of Ken. He had been a track star before his break. Withdrawal from active movement was a key sign of his acute distress.

Ken would frequently select a sound-effect record and proceed to move out his fantasies in a self-directed manner. He often took initial cues from the recorded sounds.

Recurring images and themes emerged from this work. Consistently Ken needed to conquer gigantic obstacles such as high mountains and barren deserts which called for massive strength and endurance on his part.

He struggled and labored along his hero's journey. Invariably, after a great expenditure of energy, he would reach his destination which was most often a mountain top. Usually he would look down on what lay beneath him and announce that it was not what he was looking for. He battled with themes of immortality. Often the city, or whatever he had left behind, had been destroyed. He repeatedly encountered death and rebirth.

It was clear to me that one of the major themes that Ken was working on was trust. My role was to bring the quality of trust to all of our contact. It was crucial that I remained centered in a space of unconditional love. Working from the vantage point of high indifference I experienced Ken as a being in transition, on the way to his next knowing.

As Ken became more trusting in our relationship the quality of the sessions changed. Spontaneous laughter emerged. The warm-ups became more playful and took on a flavor of indulging in forgotten childhood games.

After a month's work, a "thawing out" of the initial "frozen" quality started to be visible. This was particularly evident in Ken's increased range and appropriateness of facial expression. The changes in the resiliency of the superficial fascia of his face were clearly observable.

He allowed himself to engage in and enjoy large muscle movements where initially he had severely restricted himself to small, gestural motions. Ken began to use space more vigorously, more directly, and with increased sense of purpose. He began to claim his own power and full size. In his fear he had pulled taut his energy membrane. As he permitted greater trust his vitality expanded.

Ken became more assertive both in our sessions and with staff and peers on the unit. He began to ask for what he wanted. He began to experiment with themes of dependence and independence in the movement work before applying them to other contacts.

A running motif in our work was Ken's relationship to God. He began to come to an understanding that there was a "little piece of God" inside him and that he was seeking to become more like God. It became clearer that his images of climbing to high places were in hopes of having glimpses of spiritual experiences.

The fantasy explorations continued throughout the four months of our work. The talking we did at the end of each session suggested that he was gaining increased insights into his reality and view of the universe. His work appeared to represent a ritual of gaining mastery of self in a major transition of his life as he discovered his independent identity.

Through the therapeutic relationship Ken was able to release some archaic fears—such as his feeling he was the devil incarnate. He gained a sense of purpose and direction, and began to shift his focus towards unification. Although Ken was involved in other intense forms of psychotherapy during his hospital stay, I am convinced that transpersonal-transformational movement therapy uniquely provided him the space to give form, feeling and meaning to some of his personal metaphors and to begin to comprehend the nature of trust.

Bibliography

Dass, Ram. *The Only Dance There Is.* Garden City, New York: Anchor Books, 1974.

Derbolowsky, Gretel. "Dealing and Working with Materials in Group Analysis and with LSD 25," Hamburg, Germany. Typed manuscript, undated. Presented at British Conference on Social Psychiatry, London, 1964.

Dunbar, Flanders. *Mind and Body: Psychosomatic Medicine.* New York, Random House, 1955 (revised edition).

Golas, Thaddeus. *The Lazy Man's Guide to Enlightenment.* Palo Alto: The Seed Center, 1971.

Hillman, James. *Insearch.* New York: Charles Scribner's Sons, 1967.

Hinsie, Leland E. *The Person in the Body—An Introduction to Psychosomatic Medicine.* New York: Norton & Co., 1945.

Joy, Brugh. Seminars at Sky Hi Ranch, Lucerne Valley, California, 1976.

Laing, R.D. *The Divided Self.* Baltimore: Penguin Books, 1967.

Loeks, Kathleen Savides. Seminars on Essential Integration, an evolutionary body work. Los Angeles, 1977–8.

Maslow, Abraham, H. *The Farther Reaches of Human Nature.* New York: The Viking Press, 1971.

Roberts, Jane. *The Nature of Personal Reality: A Seth Book.* Englewood Cliffs: Prentice-Hall, Inc., 1974.

Rolf, Ida P. and Hunt, Valerie V. "Body Energetics: Structural Integration." Speech delivered at 2nd Conference on Psycho-energetics of Consciousness sponsored by Center for the Healing Arts, Los Angeles, 1975.

Russell, Douglas. "Psychosynthesis." Printed pamphlet, Los Angeles, 1977.
Schoop, Trudi. *Won't You Join the Dance? A Dancer's Essay into the Treatment of Psychosis.* Palo Alto: National Press Books, 1974.
Thomas, Lewis. *The Lives of A Cell.* New York: Viking Press, 1974.
Waelder, Robert. *Basic Theory of Psychoanalysis.* New York: International University Press, 1960.
Watson, Lyall. *Gifts of Unknown Things,* New York: Simon & Schuster, 1976.
Winer, Eileen Pittler. Seminars on Sympathetic Vibrational Magnetism, Los Angeles, 1975–8.

Section III

A COMPARATIVE ANALYSIS

Chapter 11
METHODS OF COMPARISON

Rationale

Dance therapy needs a common vocabulary. It needs a body of knowledge—a theoretical frame of reference to provide a foundation for the profession and its practice (Smallwood, Kalish, Chaiklin, 1976, p. 2).

The purpose of this comparative analysis is to move toward this goal by providing a theory of dance-movement therapy based on the understanding and integration of the essential meaning of the major theoretical approaches in use in dance-movement therapy today. A more holistic approach in relation to existing movement therapy theory is of benefit to the public (Bernstein, 1975, p. 5; Chaiklin 1968, p. 67 and 1974, p. 59; Geller, 1974, p. 3).

With the introduction of an holistic theory of dance-movement therapy dance therapists are provided with a researched explicit, common conceptual ground upon which to stand, and communicate with one another. Cross fertilization of approaches, as well as new theoretical constructs, can occur. With an holistic theory of dance-movement therapy the public is availed the possiblility for a clearer understanding of the field. The public encompasses clinical administrative staff who are in a position to hire dance therapists, fellow mental health professionals, governmental agencies and foundations capable of supporting the field, and potential clients who are in the need of a holistic body-oriented therapy. These individuals now have access to a concise discussion of the theory of dance-movement therapy.

In addition, clarification based on key fundamental concepts and hypotheses in each of the eight approaches represented in this book was made in an organized, systematic manner through a method of research which allows each of these frames of reference to reveal themsleves.

Phenomenological Method

Specifically, this comparative analysis is designed to investigate and clarify the dance therapists' experience of her conceptual frame of reference through the use of a phenomenological approach in order to obtain a fundamental holistic dance-movement therapy theory. The frame of reference chapters represent the responses of key proponents of the major approaches being taught and utilized in the field.

Each chapter was analyzed in terms of the author's response to the following basic psychotherapy theorietcal considerations:

What is the theoretical base?

How is the health-dysfunction continuum viewed and what is the method(s) utilized for its identification and evaluation?

How is dance-movement therapy viewed and what is the therapeutic process?

Phenomenology has been selected as the appropriate research methodology for this study as it encourages and allows for the clarification of experience in a way that facilitates the essence of the meaning of the ideas in question. Von Eckartsberg (1975) studied various theories phenomenologically and arrived at an "eco-psychology" which represents a synthesis of the frames of reference discussed.

Further, the more traditional scientific methodological qualities of experimental designs, are incompatible with the needs of this comparison. Quantity, although required to ascertain the major approaches,* does not lend itself to intensive qualitative scrutiny of data (Giorgi, 1971, pp. 19–20). Measurement, typically basic to all traditional scientific research, is not a needed factor here. Neither is it necessary to promulgate the assumption that the observer is somehow independent of his/her study and in no way influences its outcome. By virtue of the structuring and defining of the experimental situation, the researcher is delineating the study.

In its stead phenomenologist, Giorgi (1971, pp. 25–25) proposes the concept of participant observer. By participant it is understood that no researcher, no matter how scrupulously his/her attempts are, can ever be totally independent of the research when engaged in the study of human experience. Individuals, whether the subjects or the researchers, are continuously engaged in an interactive relationship with their experiential environment. When the scientist is engaged in his/her project, its design, implementation and interpretation; his/her influencing point of view is present and therefore must be acknowledged. This allows for his/her background experience with the subject matter to be recognized and proper perspective to be placed on the study. Thus with assumptions made explicit, the study can then utilize rather than deny or attempt to delimit the knowledge and experience in dance-movement therapy theoretical formations of the editor.

Important to note is the fact that there exists no one method for doing a phenomenological study. Phenomenological research is a generic concept delineating those studies which adhere to the philosophy of phenomenology in their methods of seeking to understand the meaning of experience. The major qualities of this kind of research are elucidated by Giorgi (1975).

The analysis of the theoretical approaches proceeded in the following manner:

Natural meaning units relating to the specific questions asked the theoretical approaches were extrapolated from the individual texts.

Each natural meaning unit consisted of varying levels of conceptual and propositional responses to the therapist's experience of her view of the proposed areas in question. The therapist's personal evolution toward the crystalization and use of the approach (genesis), her direct discussion of the concepts and theoretical formulations (theoretical model), and her description of the application of the frame and reference with an individual engaged in dance-movement therapy (case study) revealed the meaning of dance therapy theory from different vantage points. From the meaning units, the therapist's response to the questions were intuited and restated in related central themes. Thus statements which delineate the central meaning of the author-dance therapist's thematic gestalts were made in relation to the questions asked.

Situated and unsituated themes** were aquired through the structural reorganization and reduction of redundances of the related central themes of each natural meaning unit. The un-

*The decision regarding the major approaches selected for this book was based on the results of a series of surveys sponsored by the American Dance Therapy Association Ad Hoc Committee on Private Practice and Task Force Body of Knowledge Committee.

**Situated themes are statements crouched in the language of the particular approach. Unsituated themes are statements in which specific approach based language has been replaced with general language.

situated themes were accomplished by redefining in a more fundamental general language those concepts which were associated with the particular frame of reference. Restatement of each description in this way not only served as a test of the thematic statement's ability to communicate essential invariant meaning regardless of the situation into which it is transposed, but it also facilitated comparison of the experience of dance therapy theoretical frames of reference among the nine contributors. These restatements were then verified with the dance therapist-author herself to insure no loss or distortion of meaning.

Each proponent was also given an opportunity to read the unsituated themes of the other seven approaches. Each was asked to eliminate any phrasing or conceptual material which did not fit her view of her approach. The verified and clarified unsituated statements were clustered by theme and recognized by a key word, concept of assumption such as body awareness, movement improvisation, or body-mind holism. Only those themes which were either present in the chapters or agreed upon as congruent by the authors were included in the theoretical construction of a holistic frame of reference. The resultant theoretical approach then represents the common experience of the contributors view of dance-movement therapy theory based on their personal view of the approach they represented.

Chapter 12

A HOLISTIC FRAME OF REFERENCE IN DANCE-MOVEMENT THERAPY

The following represents the fundamental conceptual structure of the major frames of reference employed in the training and clinical work of dance therapists based on the responses of key proponents of the theoretical models. Important to note here is that this comparative analysis is not meant to be exhaustive in its identifying themes of dance therapy theory. Rather, it attempts to begin the task of surfacing and delineating the body of knowledge which is foundational to the field of movement therapy. It is toward this journey that this analysis has addressed itself.

Theoretical Base of Dance-movement Therapy

Holism

The individual in relation to self. The individual is viewed as an integrated unity; mind and body reflect and effect each other. Muscle tonus effects the psychic attitude and visa versa.

The individual in relation to the environment. Mind, body, organic functioning, and behavior are interwoven with the environment.

Development

Manner of Development. The individual develops in an organized sequential manner.

Learning and Memory. Developmentally related, intermeshed somatic experiences, unconscious material and conscious behavior are stored in the individual. Present experience may be influenced by and trigger past stored experience bringing past behavior to present.

Growth Process. The individual has an innate capacity for continuous growth. The individuals' natural rhythm and timing is used when engaging in growth.

Polarities. The individual has physical and psychic polarities. Utilizing the innate capacity for growth, the individual strives toward the unity of these polarities.

Formal Structural Constructs

Unconscious. The individual has an unconscious consisting of that which the individual is unaware.

Consciousness. The individual has the potential for a consciousness consisting of that which the individual is aware.

Ego. The ego is that part of the consciousness which is needed to assist in the therapy process.

Body Image. The individual has a continuous mental representation of his/her self. This representation provides an awareness of the differentiation of and optimum comfort space between self and the environment.

Health-dysfunction Continuum in Dance-movement Therapy

Formal Conceptual Propositions

Holistic unity-disunity. Health is reflected in mind-body integration; dysfunction is reflected in mind-body split and in the somatization of psychic problems.

Growth Process. Health is reflected in capacity to engage in the individual's own realization of wholeness, this entails the cooperation of the ego and the unconscious. Dysfunction is reflected in the difficulty or inability to engage in the individual's own integration process.

Experiencing the Moment. Health is viewed as the capacity to be aware of and accurately perceive present experience intra-personally, interpersonally, and in relation to life events. This entails the capacity to experience the full range of human feelings as they emerge and to be able to consciously conceptualize the experience. Lack of present involvement is reflected in sustained, habitual often developmentally related distortions of self, body image, expression, others, and of his/her being-in-the-world.

Need Satisfaction. Health and dysfunction is reflected in the degree to which an individual meets his/her needs.

Social Interaction. Health is reflected in the capacity for meaningful social interaction.

Concrete Somatic Propositions

Body: Health-dysfunction continuum is reflected somatically in the body.

Health	*Dysfunction*
Integrated unified body	Body splits
Balanced, aligned body	Imbalanced body
Normal breath flow	Dysfunctional breath flow
Natural energy flow	Body blocks

Body Movement: Health-dysfunction continuum is reflected somatically in body movement.

Health	*Dysfunction*
Adaptive range of movement qualities	Habitual non-adaptive limited range of movement qualities
Graceful coordinated integrated movements	Distorted, uncoordinated, unintegrated movements
Ability to be aware of and utilize conscious and unconscious movement	Inability to be aware of and utilize conscious and unconscious movement

Postulates Regarding the Method(s) of Identification and Evaluation of the Health-dysfunction Continuum in Dance-movement Therapy

*Health-dysfunction continuum may be identified and evaluated through the observation of body-movement along with other somatic behavior.**

*Refer to concrete somatic propositions of the health-dysfunction continuum for delineation.

Health-dysfunction continuum may be identified and evaluated through the clients verbalization primarily entailing the conscious presentations of problems and the associations to body-movement experiences.

Postulates Regarding Change: Definition of Dance-movement Therapy

Dance-movement Therapy Entails the Use of Dance-movement.

The particular use of dance-movement can include:

- Contraction-relaxation patterns
- Postural-gestural patterns
- Range of movement qualities
- Developmentally related movement
- Rhythmic dance
- Spontaneous movement/creative dance
- Thematic movement improvisations
- Unconscious symbolic body movement
- Group dance

Dance Movement Therapy Is a Process.

This process can be concerned with:

Present awareness in relation to the individual's body, intrapsychic functioning, body movement, relationship with therapist and others and in relation to the individual's history.

Exploration, experience, expression, and *identification* of conscious and unconscious material, polarities, energy blocks, and emotions.

Dance-movement Therapy Is Used for the Purpose of Integration Toward Wholeness.

This purpose may results in:

- Intrapsychic change or reorganization
- Conflict resolution
- Realization if individual's potential
- Capacity to meet ones needs
- Maintenance of present awareness
- Natural flow of energy
- Increased capacity for vitality and relaxation
- Meaningful social interaction

Summary: Dance-movement Therapy is a process entailing the use of dance-movement for awareness, expression, exploration, identification, and integration toward the experience of wholeness.

Postulates Regarding Change: Therapeutic Process in Dance-movement Therapy

Beginning Phase

Starting where the individual is in the moment, s/he may move or verbally relate experience. The therapist observes and facilitates the individual's awareness and exploration of their nonverbal behavior.

This initial process may be carried out via:

- Suggestions for sensory awareness
- Empathetic mirroring by the therapist
- Suggestions for movement improvisations
- Warm-up exercises
- Allowing space for spontaneous movement exploration

Middle Phase

Through the use of body-movement, experience of unintegrated often unconscious symbolic aspects of the individual is focused.

Through the use of body-movement, experience of the individual's strengths may, on occasion, be focused.

This experience may be facilitated via:

- Suggestions for movement improvisations via image or themes
- Allowing non-directive space for movement exploration
- Therapist moving in synchronicity or reciprosity with the individual
- Group rhythmic dance
- Verbalization before, during, or in response to movement

Final Phase

Conscious awareness via verbal associations, insight producing interpretation, and/or comments by the therapist and client/patient are made pertaining to the relationship of the unconscious material to the individual's experience of present life.

Exploration of new ways of perception, expression, and of being-in-the world through movement may also be developed.

Relationship of a Holistic Dance-movement Therapy Frame of Reference to Other Models of Psychotherapy

Medical Model

The medical model characteristically views any individual who needs psychotherapy as ill or sick. When the individual is suitably finished with therapy, they are considered to be cured. The therapeutic process is viewed as treatment and the individual as patient. Psychiatric medical institutions are often primarily concerned with symptom removal and less with in-depth psychology (Alperson, 1976; Siegler & Osmond, 1974).

It is a well known fact in the field of dance-movement therapy that aside from a few therapists engaged in private practice, the majority of dance therapists work in clinical settings which support the medical model. Important also to note is the fact that all approved graduate programs in dance therapy must provide a minimum of a six-month or seven hundred hour internship in these clinical settings (ADTA, Dance Therapy Graduate School Guidelines, 1976).

Relation to the Theoretical Base

Although the medical model would align itself with a holistic view of an individual, in practice, a different experience might be reflected. The medical orientation is to what one "has"

(Siegler, Osmond, 1974, p. 48). The dance-movement therapy model is more concerned with what one "is experiencing."

Belief in an innate capacity for continuous growth is a distinctly different orientation than a model which views an individual who could benefit from therapy as sick or abnormal.

The formal structural constructs of conscious-unconscious, ego and body-image all are not unheard of in the medical model, but have secondary importance to concepts of a biochemical and genetic orientation (Siegler, Osmond, 1974).

Relation to Health-dysfunction Continuum, Its Identification and Evaluation

Again, although those holding with the medical model would not disagree with the fundamental view of the health-dysfunction continuum, its focus is on the symptom(s) and the cure of mental illness.

Diagnosis is made, placing a label on the individual—a label which she/he sometimes wears throughout life. During the reduction process of this research, however, it became clear that the concept of a continuum between health and dysfunction was the pervasive view of the chapter contributors. Fixed labeling was not fundamentally present. Rather, behavioral descriptions that impeded or faciliated the individual's being-in-his/her-world were found to be germane.

Relation to Postulates Regarding Change

Aside from the obvious lack of focus on body-movement, the medical model physiologic view of personality seeks to cure through medical procedures. The most widely used is that of chemotherapy. The focus is the "relief of suffering."

Dance-movement Therapy is viewed as a process entailing enlarged self understanding—a process which might delve into psychic pain in order for a deeper integration to occur." Process focus is virtually not present in the medical model. The relationship between patient and therapist is no more significant than it is with any other medical relationship (Alperson, 1976). Seiger and Osmond describe this role of the psychiatrist as being potentially imbued with Aesculapian authority (Seigler, Osmond, 1974, p. 135–137). In this position physicians confer the sick or well role on individuals and prescribe remediation.

Concepts such as the mutual engagement in an individual's awareness, exploration, experience, identification, interpretation, and integration are not available when the therapist gives the advice and assumes responsibility for treatment.

Interesting to note here is the fact that in spite of the strong philosophic differences, dance therapy departments exist primarily within medical model oriented institutions. Two diverse rationales for this are that (1) some psychiatrists are trained and utilize therapeutic process approaches such as psychoanalytic, family systems (Ackerman, Jackson, Bowen, Minuchin, et al), or Sullvanian interpersonal theory or (2) other physicians may view dance therapy's use as primarily providing needed physical exercise for their patients and not as a form of psychotherapy.

Behavioral Model

Although John Watson coined the term behaviorism, the contributions of B.F. Skinner and Ivan Pavlov are considered to be the foundations of the behavioral model. Joseph Wolpe's work in reciprocal inhibition evolved from the classical conditioning model of Pavlov. In this model, the unconditioned stimulus (UCS) is coupled with a conditioned stimulus resulting in a conditioned response no longer dependent on the UCS. The Skinnerian operant conditioning model is most noticeably implemented in token economics and other reinforcement paradimes. In general this model represents a precise systematic mechanistic view of the individual, health and dysfunction and the therapeutic process based on the learning, shaping, inhibition and extinguishment of patterns of behavior (Burton, 1974; Ford & Urban, 1967; Mosey, 1970; Alperson, 1976).

Dance therapists who do not subscribe to this approach have found it particularly difficult to translate their relationship with the individual into one which would also serve the purposes of behavior modification. They may achieve the same behavioral results, but the method experientially appears to be different.

Relation to the Theoretical Base

The individual is viewed in terms of his/her behavior. Emphasis is placed on habits, operant conditioning, stimulus-response and reinforcement. This focus appears to emphasize and is in agreement with the holistic dance therapy theory view of development.

Other areas such as growth process, unconscious symbolic material, existent polarities, and holism are relevant only as they relate to target behaviors.

Relation to Health-dysfunction Continuum, Its Identification and Evaluation

Like behaviorism, dance therapy theory utilizes observation of behavior as a major tool for the purposes of identification and evaluation. However the proposition of health and dysfunction being part of a continuum is not applicable in a system in which the emphasis is placed on the existence or non-existence of a pattern of behavior.

Target behavior is viewed primarily within an external social context. Thus the dance therapy proposition of health reflecting the capacity for meaningful social interaction would be in accordance with behaviorists. However, the idea that dysfunctional behavior is just a bad habit, appears to be too reductionistic for basic movement therapy theory. The subtitles of intrapsychic conflict and disunity are not of concern in and of themselves.

Relation to Postulates Regarding Change

The behavior therapist views his/her therapy as the teaching of new, more appropriate behavior to the client or patient. The therapist assigns behaviors, prescribes rehearsals, and trains the client to engage in specific behaviors. Like the therapist engaged in the medical model, the relationship is authoritarian in nature. The therapy is process oriented only within the specific context of the altering or extinguishment of target behavior. Structure is maintained.

Unlike dance therapy theory, awareness, exploration, identification and integration do not occur in a holistic context, but only in relation to the behavior vis a vis the environment. Techniques which are designed to elicit unconscious symbolic material and developmentally related experiences are not, therefore, in and of themselves relevant.

Exploration of new ways of responding to an individual's life are used, but only in specific relationships to the pattern to be extinguished. Dance therapy process may, at times, be as specific but may also run the gamut to more general application.

Growth Model

The growth model seems to resonate most with the fundamental structure concepts of dance-movement therapy theoretical frame of reference. Abraham Maslow's (1954) concept of self actualization, human potential, and the on-going process of growth, are strongly represented in the results of this investigation. The focus on the use of experience within the therapeutic process is typical of the humanistic-growth model and intrinsic in dance therapy (Murphy 1958, 1972; Murray, 1962).

Relation to Theoretical Base

The individual being viewed as an interrelated whole was emphasized and promulgated by the humanists. (This emphasis has engaged many growth models in the use of the body, non-verbal communication, and a foucs on the somatizations of conflict.) The individual's innate capacity for continuous growth is reflected in the name of the model itself.

Polarities and their experience are one of the major foci of Gestalt therapy as well as other specific approaches. Finally the formal structures, conceptualized by Freud remain part of the backbone of any psychodynamic approach including those considered to be growth models.

Relation to Health-dysfunction Continuum, Its Identification and Evaluation

Health and dysfunction are viewed as a continuum within the humanistic approaches. An individual is not labeled; rather, behaviors resulting from interpersonal environmental experience are focused upon. The possibilities of choice are therefore available to the client.

The degree to which integration is reflected in mind-body interrelationship is a view which resonates with humanists. A great deal of emphasis is placed on the capacity to experience the moment. Existential psychologist Rollo May (1953, 1958, 1960), Fritz Perls (1951), as well as other conceptualizers and contributors to humanistic-growth models consider this proposition as fundamental to their approach.

Relation to Postulates Regarding Change

The humanists' view of the therapeutic relationship with a client is participatory in nature. Rogers (1965), speaks of empathetic reflection; Chace's use of reflective recreating is clearly the body movement analogue.

Growth models are process oriented. Concepts such as awareness, exploration, experience, and identification are basic to therapy.

Starting where the individual is reciprocated in the "here-now" orientation of Gestalt, and existential-phenomenological approaches.

Body awareness in the form of sentence completions such as, "Now I am aware of . . . " or "Now I am feeling . . . " are often used in the development of the figure in Gestalt Therapy. In this way, Gestalt and other humanistically oriented growth models, encourage bringing unconscious unintegrated material into conscious awareness.

Rogers provides an environment of "unconditional positive regard" for the free expression of repressed negative and ambivalent feelings. The therapeutic relationship promulgates a more independent nature insuring that the individual's own personal responsibility is active.

Elaine Seigel's psychoanalytic orientation of movement from great dependence to independence would be in accordance with the direction of the therapist—individual relationship.

Conscious integration through insight and understanding is as intrinsic to the growth model as it is to the dance therapy model.

Finally, exploration of new ways of perception, expression, and of being-in-the-world is built into Rogerian client-centered therapy (1965) and often a finishing experiment to a completed Gestalt (Polster & Polster, 1973)

Emerging Reflections

Although there exists a common fundamental base among all the major approaches presented in this book, they, nonetheless, have their own uniqueness. It is to the relationship of their distinctness to the dance therapist that I wish to direct these final statements.

As studies to date have indicated, no one frame of reference is more effective or efficient than any other (Mosey, 1970; Lindzey, 1954; Ford and Urban, 1963); the dance-movement therapist's comfort or syntonicity with the theoretical approach then becomes highly important.

Through my years of training graduate students in a variety of dance therapy models, certain relationships to the students personal psychology and the skills required by some of the approaches began to be drawn.

Carl Jung's psychological typology seems to clarify this phenomenon. Jung intuited through his analytic work with individuals that there existed certain basic adaptations to life and that some people favor certain viewpoints and others, other orientations.

There are those who view their world from a rational *thinking* orientation. These individual's have highly honed analytic ability. Thinking that is connected to objective facts or experience or to general traditional ideas inferred from external phenomena is considered as extroverted. This is the typical empirical scientific orientation to existence. When the objective data is subjectified i.e., when the thoughts start from the subject and are directed to subjective ideas, the orientation is introverted.

Thinking types view the world within an historical progression. Life is seen as a linear process evolving from past existence. These individuals often have a clear mapped out delineation of their future as well.

The opposite rational orientation is that of *feeling*. Individuals in whom this is a primary means of relating are more concerned with judging how something feels rather than an analysis of its components. They engage in valuations of experience. Extrovert feelers are influenced by and sensitive to the objects of society's values or emotions. The introvert individual determines his/her feelings subjectively and internally.

On the other side are the orientations concerned with perceiving. Those whose reference point is sensation, exist in a present orientation to life. Extrovert sensors have an acute sense of the moment. They do not seem to need to place the present in any particular temporal context. Introvert sensation psychologies often have a heightened awareness of their somatic internal functioning. Those of the sensation orientation do not relate well with anything that is tinged with an unknown, unseeable area of transpersonal psychology.

Sensations opposite: introvert intuitors, however, bask in symbols, myths, and the empirically unknown. These individuals along with extrovert intuitors rely on hunches emerging from the unconscious. Extrovert intuitors often have an excellent sense about what will happen next in relation to others or situational events.

Now what do these psychological orientations have to do with a dance therapists' frame of reference? Simply that different orientations seem to suit the utilization of different theoretical approaches.

For example, Freud was clearly a thinking type. Psychoanalytic therapy makes strong use of analytic interpretation and an awareness of the relationship of the individual's past to his/her present state. Psychodyanmic and Adlerian approaches make use of the thinking function as well.

Marian Chace, on the other hand, was not interested in engaging in analytic interpretations. She has been considered to have worked primarily out of a feeling—intuitive orientation.

Gestalt Therapy, with its focus on present awareness requires more of a sensation orientation to therapy. Perls was considered to be a feeling-sensation type. It was Hefferline and Goodman who were concerned with theory building (requiring a thinking function). Perls was considered to be the "showman."*

Analytic psychology necessitates the use of Jung's psychological orientation, that of introvert intuition. In order to trust and follow an individual's unconscious, the therapist would have to trust his/her own intuitive hunches. Likewise, any engagement in transpersonal psychotherapy would require an active intuitive process.

From tests such as the Myer-Briggs which delineate an individual's psychological orientation, it appears that both students and dance therapy clinicians seem to integrate and resonate more with the theroetical approaches which suit their primary mode of psychological orientation.**

Lest a holistic view of the individual is lost. It would seem important to note here that all these orientations are present within each persons psychology; in most instances one or more dominates in early adulthood. Jung believed that often, as the individual reaches around thirty-five years of age there seems to be a surge of energy toward psychological unity and shadow or undeveloped functions become more figural, availing the possibility of integration to transpire.

To state that these theoretical approaches require only the use of one orientation or another would, of course, do them an injustice as well. Thinking analytically, feeling empathetically, sensing with awareness, and intuiting with access to the universal pool of knowledge are all needed if the dance therapist is to enrich his/her chosen theoretical approach with humanity.

*Lecture-discussion from Isadore Fromm, 1975.

**Based on pilot study at Antioch-New England Graduate School, 1978.

Bibliography

Adler, Alfred. *The Practice and Theory of Individual Psychology*. New York: Harcourt Brace, 1924.

Alperson, Erma. Deviant Behavior in Relation to the Practice of Psychotherapy. Unpublished handout, 1976.

Alperson, Erma. Movement Therapy—A Theoretical Framework. In Donelan, Fran, Ed., *Writings on Body Movement and Communication,* Columbia: ADTA, Vol III, 1973.

American Dance Therapy Association Newsletter, Columbia: ADTA, 3 1968–10 1976.

American Dance Therapy Association Proceedings Fifth Annual Conference, Columbia: ADTA, 1970

American Dance Therapy Association Proceedings Third Annual Conference, Columbia: ADTA, 1968.

Bartenieff, Irmgard. Exploring Interaction Through Ritual Structure. *Therapeutic Process: Movement as Integration,* Columbia: ADTA, 1974, 118–122.

Bartenieff, Irmgard. Contribution of Effort/Shape to Technique & Style in Dance. *Proceedings of Ninth Annual Conference on Creative Teaching of Dance,* New York: 1965.

Bartenieff, Irmgard, and Davis, Martha. Effort-Shape Analysis of Movement: The Unity of Expression and Function. *Research Approaches to Movement and Personality* is one of a series entitled *Body Movement: Perspectives in Research,* New York: Arno Press, 1975.

Bartenieff, Irmgard, Davis, Martha and Paulay, Forrestine. *Four Adaptations of Effort Theory in Research and Teaching.* New York: Dance Notation Bureau, 1970.

Bartenieff, Irmgard, and Paulay, Forrestine. Choreometrics Profiles. In Lomax, Alan, *Folk Song Style and Culture.* Washington, D.C.: American Association for the Advancement of Science, Publication No. 88, 1968.

Bartenieff, Irmgard, and Paulay, Forrestine. Research in Anthropology: A Study of Dance Styles in Primitive Cultures. *Research in Dance: Problems and Possibilities.* New York: Committee on Research in Dance (CORD), 1967.

Barton, Anthony. *Three World of Therapy.* Palo Alto: National Book Press, 1974.

Bernstein, Penny. Recapitulation of Ontogeny: A Theoretical Approach in Dance Movement Therapy. *Dance Therapist in Dimension: Depth and Diversity,* Columbia, ADTA, 1973.

Bernstein, Penny. *Theory & Methods in Dance Movement Therapy.* Dubuque, Iowa: Kendall/Hunt Publishing Company, 1975.

Bernstein, Penny and Bernstein, Lawrence. A Conceptualization of Group Dance-Movement Therapy as Ritual Process. *Writings on Body Movement and Communication Monograph,* 1973 (Serial No. 3).

Bion, Wilfred. *Experiences in Groups.* New York: Basic Books, 1961.

Burton, Arthur, Ed., *Operational Theories of Personality.* New York: Brunner/Mazel Publ., 1974.

Campbell, Joseph, Ed., *The Portable Jung.* New York: Penguin Books, 1971.

Canner, Norma. . . . *And a Time to Dance.* Boston: Beacon Press, 1968.

Chaiklin, Harris. Research and the Development of a Profession. *American Dance Therapy Association Proceedings,* 1968, 64–74.

Chaiklin, Harris. Multiple Theoretical Perspectives in Interpreting Behavior. *Therapeutic Process: Movement As Integration,* Columbia: ADTA, 1974, 48–60.

Chaiklin, Harris, Ed., *Marian Chace: Her Papers.* Columbia: ADTA, 1975.

Chaiklin, Sharon. Dance Therapy. *American Handbook of Psychiatry,* New York: Basic Books, 1975.

Chaiklin, Sharon, Kalish, Beth and Smallwood, Joan. A Position Paper. Paper presented at the Tenth Annual American Dance Therapy Association Conference, Washington, D.C., October, 1976.

*Dance Therapist in Dimension: Depth and Diversity, Proceedings of the Eighth Annual Conference,*Columbia: ADTA, 1973b.

Dance Therapy: Roots and Extensions, Proceedings of Sixth Annual Conference of the American Dance Therapy Association, Columbia: ADTA, 1971b.

Darwin, Charles. *The Expression of Emotions in Man and Animals.* New York: Appleton Publishers, 1873.

Davis, Charles. *The Expression of Emotions in Man and Animals*. New York: Appleton Publishers, 1873.
Davis, Martha A. *Understanding Body Movement: An Annotated Bibliogrphy*. New York: Arno Press, 1972.
Dell, Cecily. *A Primer of Movement Description*. Dance Notation Bureau, 1970.
Donelan, Fran, Ed., *Writings on Body Movement and Communication,* Columbia: ADTA, Vols. I–III, 1971a, 1972a, 1973a (Monograph).
Duncan, Isadora. *My Life*. New York: Liverright Paperbound Edition, 1972.
Erickson, Eric. *Childhood and Society*. New York: W.W. Norton and Co., 1963.
Espenak, Liljan. Trance and Ecstasy in Dance Therapy. *Therapeutic Process: Movement as Integration,* Columbia: ADTA, 1974b, 103–117.
Fletcher, Diane. The Use of Movement and Body Experience in Therapy. *Therapeutic Process: Movement as Integration,* Columbia, ADTA, 1974.
Freud, Anna. *Normality and Pathology in Childhood*. New York: International University Press, 1966.
Freud, Sigmund. *An Outline of Psychoanalysis*. New York: Norton, 1949.
Ford, Donald and Hugh Urban. *Systems of Psychotherapy*. New York: John Wiley & Sons, Inc. 1967
Fourth Annual Conference Proceedings. Columbia: ADTA, 1969.
Geller, Jesse. Dance Therapy as Viewed by a Psychotherapist. *Writings on Body Movement and Communication Monograph,* 1973–4 (Serial No. 3)
Giorgi, Amedeo. *Psychology as a Human Science*. New York: Harper and Row Pub., 1970.
Giorgi, Amedeo. *Psychology as a Human Science: A Phenomenologically Based Approach*. New York: Holt, Rinehart, and Winston, Inc., 1975.
Giorgi, Amedeo, William Fischer, and Rolf Von Eckartsbert, Eds., *Duquesne Studies in Phenomenological Psychology Vol. I*. Pittsburgh: Duquesne University Press, 1971.
Giorgi, Amedeo, Fischer, E. Murray, Ed., *Duquesne Studies in Phenomenological Psychology, Vol. II*. Pittsburgh: Duquesne University Press, 1975.
Hartman, Heinz. *Ego Psychology and the Problem of Adaptation,* New York: International University Press, 1958.
Jung, Carl G., Ed., *Memories, Dreams and Reflections*. New York: Vintage Books, 1961.
Jung, Carl G., Ed., *Man and His Symbols*. London: Aldus Books Limited, 1964.
Jung, Carl G., Ed., *On the Nature of the Psyche*. Princeton: Princeton University Press, 1973.
Katz, Richard. The Painful Ecstasy of Healing. *Psychology Today*. December, 1976.
Keen, Ernest. *A Primer in Phenomenological Psychology*. New York: Hole, Rinehart and Winston, Inc., 1975.
Laban, Rudolf. *The Mastery of Movement*. London: MacDonald & Evans, 1960.
Laban, Rudolf, with Lawrence, F.C., *Effort*. New York: Dance Horizons, 1947.
Latner, Joel. *The Gestalt Therapy Book*. New York: Julian Press, Inc., 1973.
Lefco, Helene. *Dance Therapy: Narrative Case Histories of Therapy Sessions with Six Patients*. Chicago: Nelson-Hall Co., 1974.
Lomax, Alan, Ed., *Folk Song Style and Culture*. Washington: AAAS Pub. 88, 1960.
May, Rollo. *Man's Search for Himself*. New York: Dell Pub. Co., 1953.
May, Rollo. *Existential Psychology*. New York: Random House, 1960
May, Rollo. *Love and Will*. New York: Dell Pub. Co., 1969.
May, Rollo. *Power and Innocence*. New York: Dell Pub. Co., 1972.
May, Rollo, Angel, Ernst, and Ellenberger, Henri. *Existence: A New Dimension in Psychiatry and Psychology*. New York: Simon and Schuster, 1958.
Maslow, A.H., *Motivation and Personality*. New York: Harper Bros., 1954.
Meerloo, Joose Am., *The Dance from Ritual to Rock and Roll-Ballet to Ballroom*. Philadelphia: Chilton Co., 1960.
Mosey, Anne. *Three Frames of Reference for Mental Health*. Thorofare: Charles B. Slack, Inc., 1970.
Murphy, Gardner. *Human Potentials*. New York: Basic Books, 1958.
Murphy, Gardner and Konack, Joseph. *Historical Introduction to Modern Psychology*. New York: Harcourt Brace Jonanovich, Inc., 1972.
Murray, H.A., *Explorations in Personality*. New York: Science Ed., 1962.
Perls, Frederick, Hefferline, Ralph, and Goodman, Paul. *Gestalt Therapy*. New York: Dell Publishing Co. Inc., 1951.

Polster, Erving and Polster, Miriam. *Gestalt Therapy Integrated.* New York: Brunner/Mazel, 1973.
Rapport, D., *The Organization and Pathology of Thought.* New York: Columbia University Press, 1951.
Reca, Maralia. Pheomenological Method: Principles and Development in Dance Therapy. *What Is Dance Therapy Really? Proceedings of Seventh Annual Conference.* Columbia: ADTA, 1972.
Reich, Wilhelm. *Character Analysis.* New York: Farrar, Straus Girous, 1970.
Ridgeway, William. *The Dramas and Dramatic Dances of Non-European Races.* New York: Benjamin Blom, Inc., 1964.
Rogers, Carl. *Client-Centered Therapy.* Boston: Houghton Mifflin Co., 1965.
Rosen, Elizebeth. *Dance in Psychotherapy.* New York: Teachers College Press, Columbia University, 1957 (out of print).
Sachs, Curt. *World History of Dance.* New York: W.W. Norton and Co., 1963.
Second Annual Conference Proceedings. Columbia: ADTA, 1967.
Schilder, Paul. *The Image and Appearance of the Human Body.* New York: International Universities Press, Inc., 1950.
Schmais, Claire. Historical Perspective. In Mason, Kathleen, Ed., *Dance Therapy: Focus on Dance VII.* Washington: National Education Association, 1974.
Schoop, Trudi. *Won't You Join the Dance: A Dancer's Essay into the Treatment of Psychosis.* Palo Alto: National Press, 1974.
Siegel, Elaine V. Movement therapy as a psychotherapeutic tool. *Journal of The American Psychoanalytic Association,* 21: 333–343, 1973.
Siegler, Miriam and Humphrey Osmond. *Models of Madness, Models of Medicine.* New York: Harper & Row Publishers, 1974.
Stevick, Emily L. An Empirical Investigation of the Experience of Anger. In Amedeo Giorgi, William F. Fischer, E. Rolf Von Eckartsberg (Eds.). *Duquesne Studies in Phenomenological Psychology: Volume I.* Pittsburgh: Duquesne University Press, 1971.
Sullivan, H.S. *The Interpersonal Theory of Psychiatry.* New York: Norton Press, 1953.
Therapeutic Process: Movement as Integration, Proceedings of the Ninth Annual Conference. Columbia: ADTA, 1974.
Von Eckartsberg, Rolf. The Eco-Psychology of Motivational Theory and Research. In A. Giorgi, C. Fischer, & E. Murray (Eds.). *Duquesne Studies in Phenomenological Psychology Volume II.* Pittsburgh: Duquesne University Press, 1975.
What Is Dance Therapy Really? Proceedings of the Seventh Annual Conference. Columbia: ADTA, 1972b.
Whitmont, Edward. *The Symbolic Quest.* New York: Harper Colophon Books, 1969.
Wolman, Benjamin, Ed. *Dictionary of Behavioral Science.* New York: Van Nostrand Reinhold Co., 1973.

Index